Evi... cine

Finding and a... patient care

The... nd,
A...

Concept development and writing by Janet Salisbury, Biotext, Canberra, Australia

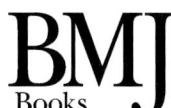

BMJ
Books

BMJ Books is an imprint of the BMJ Publishing Group

First published in 2003
by BMJ Books, BMA House, Tavistock Square
London WC1H 9JR

www.bmjbooks.com

British Library Cataloguing in Publication Data

A catalogue record for this book is available from the British Library

ISBN 0 7279 1821 4

This workbook has been developed from workshop handouts used at evidence-based medicine workshops run by the Centre for Evidence-Based Practice, Centre for General Practice, The University of Queensland. Its development was supported by the Australian Department of Health and Ageing under the Primary Health Care Research Evaluation and Development Strategy.

Production management by Biotext, Canberra
Design by Peter Nolan, Clarus Design, Canberra
Cartoons by Ian Sharpe, Canberra

Printed and bound in Spain by Graphycems, Navarra

Introduction to this workbook

Medical practitioners, particularly GPs, are overloaded with information. They simply cannot keep up with reading all the scientific literature and other information that arrives on their desk every week. Even when they have time to read some of it, it is difficult to identify which information will be most useful in clinical practice and to recall the most up-to-date findings when they need them.

But every day doctors encounter questions that need to be answered in order to make the best decisions about patient care. This is where 'evidence-based medicine' (EBM) comes in. The aim of this workbook is to introduce general practitioners and other health care professionals to the concept of EBM and to show them simple methods to find and use the best evidence to answer their clinical questions.

The workbook is practical and interactive, and will develop your skills in:

- asking clinical questions
- searching for answers
- using the answers to make clinical decisions.

At the end of this workbook, we hope that you will feel confident that you can find the best quality evidence for almost any clinical question that comes your way and, with a little practice, use it to improve your clinical practice, all within a few minutes.

How to use this workbook

This workbook has been based on the evidence-based medicine workshops run by the Centre for Evidence-Based Practice and Centre for General Practice, University of Queensland and contains information and exercises to help you learn how to use evidence-based medicine (EBM) in your clinical practice.

The workbook is divided into three main parts:

Part 1 (purple) contains an introduction to EBM and some clinical examples to show how it can be applied.

Part 2 (blue) describes the practical application of EBM. It is subdivided into five modules, each describing an important stage in the EBM process (how to formulate a question, how to track down the best evidence, how to critically appraise the evidence, how to apply the evidence and how to evaluate your progress).

Part 3 (yellow) contains information on useful internet sites and EBM resources and a number of useful articles for further reading.

If you attend one of our workshops, you will find that this workbook contains all the information that will be presented during the workshop. This means that you do not need to worry about writing down a lot of notes or copying down slides. Just relax and concentrate on the sessions. There are spaces in the kit for you to write down information during the interactive sessions and record the results of your EBM activities during the day.

The workbook has also been designed as a plain English resource document for anyone who is interested in learning more about EBM to study at their leisure or share with colleagues in small group training sessions.

In either case, we hope that you find it useful.

So that we can improve the workbook in future editions, please provide us with your feedback.

Contents

Part 1

Introduction to evidence-based medicine

EBM

What is evidence-based medicine?

Clinical practice is about making choices. Shall I order a test? Should I treat the patient? What should I treat them with? The decision depends on the doctor's knowledge, skills and attitudes, and on what resources and tests are available. The patient's concerns, expectations and values also need to be taken into account.

The term 'evidence-based medicine' (EBM) was first used by a Canadian, David Sackett and his collegues at McMaster University in Ontario, Canada in the early 1990s. They have subsequently refined the definition of EBM as integrating the best research evidence with clinical expertise and patient values to achieve the best possible patient management. EBM is about trying to improve the quality of the information on which decisions are based. It helps practitioners to avoid 'information overload' but, at the same time, to find and apply the most useful information.

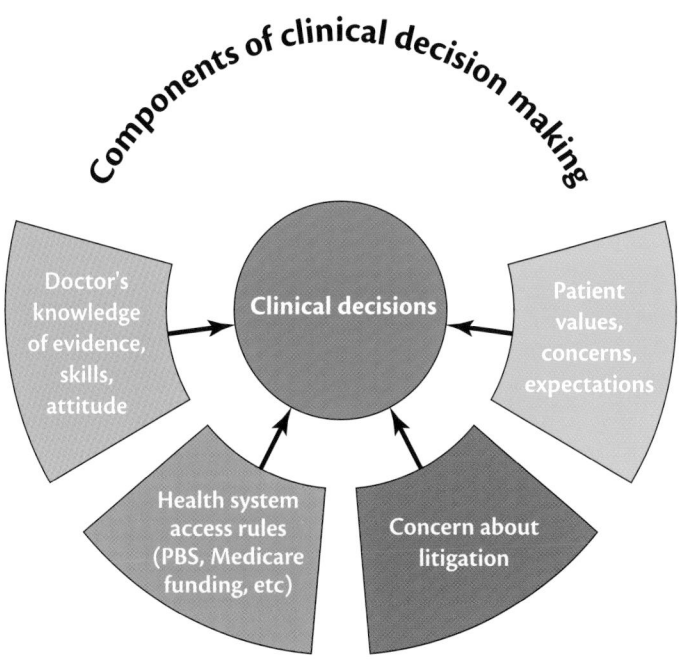

Components of clinical decision making

EBM, which has largely replaced the older term 'clinical epidemiology', is sometimes also called 'evidence-based practice'. This latter term highlights the important point that the 'evidence' that we are talking about is empirical evidence about what actually works or doesn't work in practice. It is not scientific evidence for a mechanism of action (such as a biochemical pathway, physiological effect or anatomical feature). Many factors affect the outcomes of medical activities: the underlying mechanism is only one of them. EBM is about actual clinical outcomes.

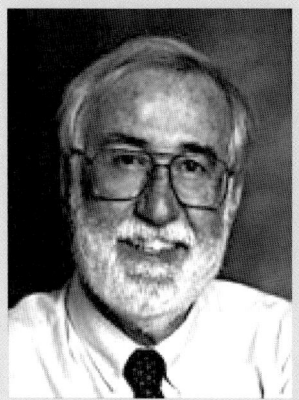

" … the integration of **best research evidence** with **clinical expertise** and **patient values**"

– Dave Sackett

Sackett DL, Stranss SE, Richardson WS *et al.* *Evidence-Based Medicine. How to practice and reach EBM*. Edinburgh: Churchill Livingstone, 2000.
Photograph reproduced with permission.

Steps in EBM

EBM uses a series of steps:

1. Formulate an answerable question.

2. Track down the best evidence of outcomes available.

3. Critically appraise the evidence (ie find out how good it is).

4. Apply the evidence (integrate the results with clinical expertise and patient values).

5. Evaluate the effectiveness and efficiency of the process (to improve next time).

Why do we need EBM?

Unfortunately, there is a large information gap between research and clinical practice. Because so much research is published all the time, clinicians understandably are unaware of most of it, or do not have the 'tools' to assess its quality. Researchers, on the other hand, do not understand the information needs of clinicians and continue to present their work in a way that is not easily accessible to busy practitioners. In 1972, British epidemiologist Archie Cochrane highlighted the fact that most treatment-related decisions were based on an ad hoc selection of information from the vast and variable quality scientific literature, on expert opinion, or, worse of all, on trial and error.

Professor Archie Cochrane was a medical researcher in the UK who contributed to the development of epidemiology as a science. In an influential book published in 1972 (Effectiveness and Efficiency), he drew attention to the great collective ignorance at that time about the effects of health care. He recognised that doctors did not have ready access to reliable reviews of available evidence. In a 1979 article he said:

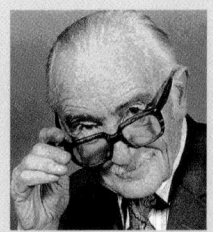

'It is surely a great criticism of our profession that we have not organised a critical summary, by speciality or subspeciality, adapted periodically, of all relevant randomised controlled trials.'

References:

Cochrane AL (1972). Effectiveness and Efficiency. Random Reflections on Health Services, Nuffield Provincial Hospital Trust, London (reprinted in 1989 in association with the British Medical Journal).
Cochrane AL (1979). 1931–1971: A critical review, with particular reference to the medical profession. In: Medicines for the Year 2000, Office of Health Economics, London.

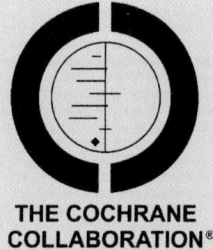

THE COCHRANE COLLABORATION®

The Cochrane Collaboration was found in response to Cochrane's call for systematic, up-to-date reviews of all relevant randomised controlled trials of health care. In the early 1990s, funds were provided by the UK National Health Service to establish a Cochrane Centre in Oxford. The approach was further outlined at an international meeting organised by the New York Academy of Sciences in 1993 and at the first Cochrane Colloquium in October 1993, when 'The Cochrane Collaboration' was founded.

http://www.cochrane.org

Cochrane logo produced with permission from The Cochrane Collaboration

Cochrane proposed that researchers and practitioners should collaborate internationally to systematically review all the best clinical trials (that is, randomised controlled trials, or RCTs), specialty by specialty. His ideas were gradually taken up during the 1980s by Iain Chalmers and one of the first areas of clinical practice to be reviewed in this way was care during pregnancy and childbirth. Systematic reviews of RCTs of different aspects of obstetric care soon showed some anomalies between the clinical trial evidence and established practice. This highlighted the gaps that existed between research and clinical practice and started to convince some doctors of the benefits of an evidence-based approach to bridge this gap.

This work has been continued though the international 'Cochrane Collaboration', which publishes systematic reviews of RCTs electronically in the Cochrane Library of Systematic Reviews. This database, which we will be looking at in detail later in the workshop, is available free online in many countries:
http://www.cochrane.org and follow the prompts.

CORTICOSTEROIDS FOR PRETERM BIRTH

1972
A RCT was reported showing improved outcomes for preterm babies when mothers were given a short course of corticosteroid before the birth.

1972–89
Six more RCTs were published which all confirmed 1972 findings.

During this time, most obstetricians were still unaware that corticosteroid treatment was so effective and so did not treat women about to give birth early with corticosteroids.

1989
First systematic review published.

1989–91
Seven more studies reported.

Corticosteroid treatment reduces the odds of babies dying from complications of immaturity by 30 to 50% but thousands of babies have died or suffered unnecessarily since 1972 because doctors did not know about the effectiveness of the treatment.

The flecainide story

The history of the use of the drug flecainide to treat heart attacks in the United States in the 1980s is a dramatic example of the gap between research and clinical practice, and the reliance on evidence of a mechanism rather than an outcome. In 1979, the inventor of the defibrillator, Bernard Lown, pointed out in an address to the American College of Cardiology that one of the biggest causes of death was heart attack, particularly among young and middle-aged men (20–64-year-olds). People had a heart attack, developed arrhythmia and died from the arrhythmia. He suggested that a 'safe and long-acting antiarrhythmic drug that protects against ventricular fibrillation' would save millions of lives.

In response to this challenge, a paper was published in the New England Journal of Medicine introducing a new drug called flecainide — a local anaesthetic derivative that suppresses arrhythmia. The paper described a study in which patients who had just had heart attacks randomly received placebo or flecainide and were then switched from one to the other (a cross-over trial). The researchers counted the number of preventricular contractions (PVCs) as a measure of arrhythmias. The patients on flecainide had fewer PVCs than the patients on placebo. When the flecainide patients were 'crossed over' to the placebo, the PVCs increased again.

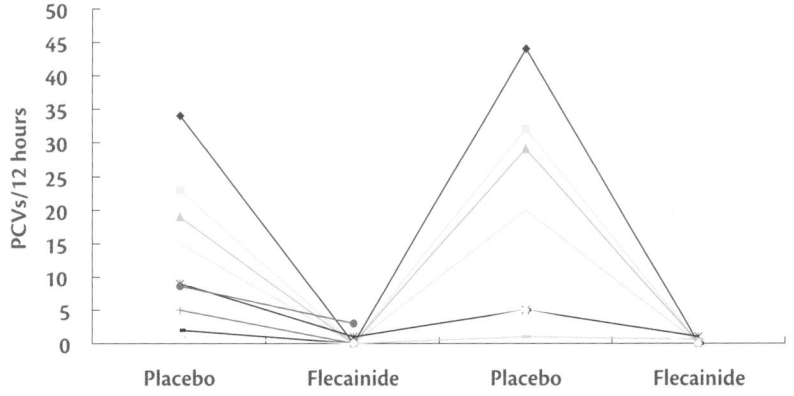

**Suppression of arrythmias in 9 patients
(PVCs = preventricular contractions)**

The conclusion was straightforward: flecainide reduces arrythmias and arrythmias cause heart attacks (the mechanism); therefore, people who have had heart attacks should be given flecainide. The results were published in the New England Journal of Medicine and flecainide was approved by the United States Food and Drug Adminstration and became fairly standard treatment for heart attack in the United States (although it did not catch on in Europe or Australia).

Almost immediately after the first trials were complete, however, other researchers had started gathering information on the survival of the patients (the outcome) instead of the PVC rate (the mechanism). This showed that over the 18 months following treatment, more than 10% of people who were given flecainide died, which was double the rate of deaths among a placebo group. In other words, despite a perfectly good mechanism for the usefulness of flecainide (it reduces arrhythmias), the drug was clearly toxic and, overall, did much more harm than good.

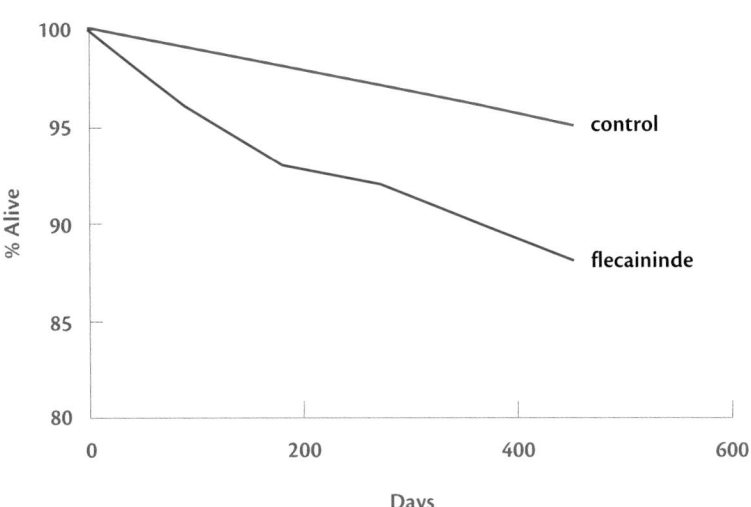

Cardiac arrythmia suppression trial (CAST)

Unfortunately, because the initial studies had been widely published in medical texts, it was a long time before doctors caught up with the subsequent poor outcome data, which did not attract as much attention. Meanwhile, about 200,000 people were being treated with flecainide in the United States by 1989. Based on the trial evidence, this would have caused tens of thousands of additional heart attack deaths due to the use of flecainide. Although there was published information, doctors were systematically killing people with flecainide because they did not know about the good quality outcome-based research.

What does the flecainide example tell us?

In the flecainide example, the initial research was widely disseminated because it was based on a traditional mechanistic approach to medicine and because it offered a 'cure'. The subsequent outcomes research may not have been widely disseminated because it was counterintuitive and negative in terms of a potential treatment. Doctors continued to prescribe flecainide because they believed that it worked. They did not know that they needed to look for further information.

Overall, the flecainide story raises two important issues:

- We need a better way to find information, even when we do not know that we need it. In other words, up-to-date, good-quality research findings need to be available to all medical practitioners on a routine basis.

- The type of research is important. We must move away from a traditional mechanistic approach and look for empirical evidence of effectiveness using a clinically relevant outcome (eg survival, improved quality of life).

References (flecainide):

Anderson JL, Stewart JR, Perry BA et al (1981). Oral flecainide acetate for the treatment of ventricular arrhythmias. New England Journal of Medicine 305:473–477.

Echt DS, Liebson PR, Mitchell LB et al (1991). Mortality and morbidity in patients receiving ecainide, flecainide, or placebo. The Cardiac Arrythmia Suppression Trial. New England Journal of Medicine 324: 781–788.

Moore TJ (1995). Deadly Medicine, Simon and Schuster, New York.

So much evidence, so little time

Doctors need to be linked to the medical research literature in a way that allows them to routinely obtain up-to-date, outcomes-based information. However, most medical practitioners, particularly GPs, are overloaded with information. Unsolicited information received though the mail alone can amount to kilograms per month and most of it ends up in the bin.

The total number of RCTs published has increased exponentially since the 1940s. A total of 20,000 trials are published each year (with over 300,000 in total) and approximately 50 new trials are published every day. Therefore, to keep up to date with RCTs alone, a GP would have to read one study report every half hour, day and night. In addition to RCTs, about 1000 papers are also indexed daily on MEDLINE from a total of about 5000 journal articles published each day.

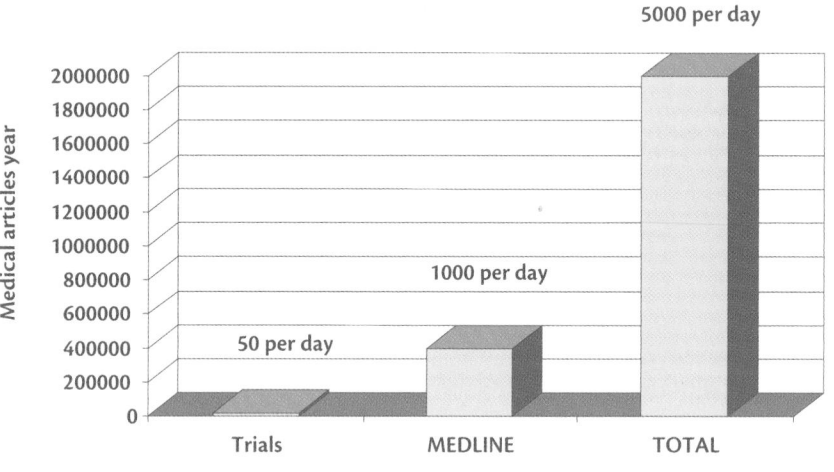

The amount of medical research

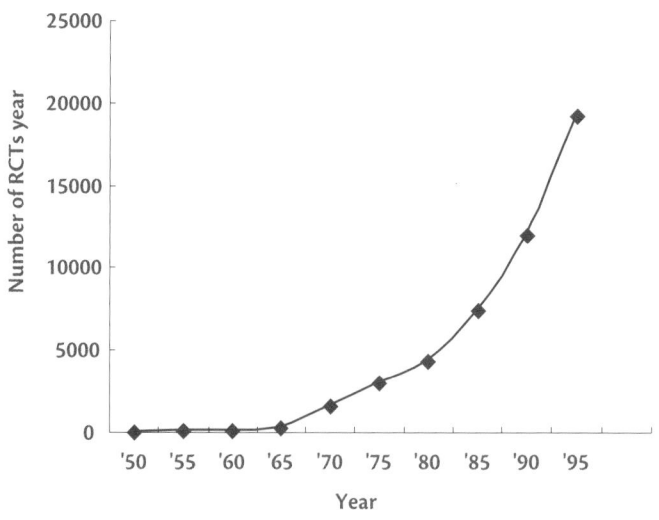

'Kill as few patients as possible'

A book by physician and medical humorist Oscar London called 'Kill as Few Patients as Possible' gives a set of 'rules' for clinical practice.

Rule 31 offers some advice on how to keep up to date with medical research:

'Review the world literature fortnightly'.

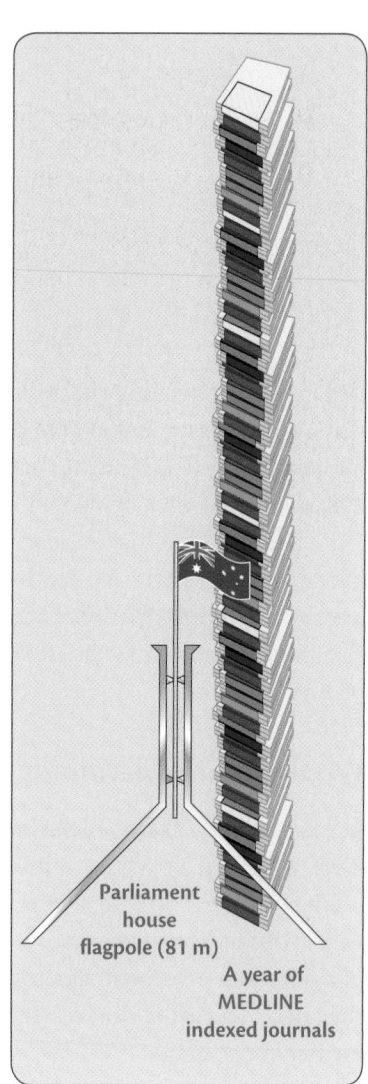

Parliament house flagpole (81 m)

A year of MEDLINE indexed journals

At best, most GPs give a selective sample of the literature a cursory review, but very little is properly assessed and almost none influences what they do in practice.

Doctors may feel guilty, anxious or inadequate because of this (see the JASPA criteria), but it is not their fault — there is just too much of it. There needs to be a better way.

JASPA criteria
(journal associated score of personal angst)

Can you answer these five simple questions:

J: Are you ambivalent about renewing your **journal** subscriptions?

A: Do you feel **anger** towards particular authors?

S: Do you use journals to help you **sleep**?

P: Are you surrounded by piles of **periodicals**?

A: Do you feel **anxious** when another one comes through the letterbox?

Score (Yes = 1; No =0):
0   anyone who scores zero is probably a liar!
1–3   normal range
>3   sick, at risk for 'polythenia gravis' and related conditions

Modified from: Polythenia gravis: the downside of evidence-based medicine. British Medical Journal (1995) 311:1666–1668.

How do doctors try to overcome information overload?

Write down some education activities that you and your organisation engage in and how much time you spend on them.

Your education activities	How much time do you spend on each?

You have probably included a selection of activities including attending lectures and conferences, reading journals, textbooks and clinical practice guidelines, electronic searching, clinical attachments and small group learning.

You may also have included talking to colleagues or specialists. But everyone has the same problem of keeping up to date and your colleagues may be out of date or just plain wrong. If they have got the information from somewhere else, you need to know where they got it so that you can check how good it is. Textbooks are always about 5–10 years out of date.

Faced with all the alternatives, how do you actually choose what to do in your continuing education time? If you are honest, your choice probably depends on what you are already most interested in rather than what you don't know about.

Continuing medical education (CME) has been a mainstay of doctors' professional development but no-one has ever shown that it works. When doctors choose their courses, they choose things that they think they need to know about. But as we have seen, the most important information is what they don't know they need! We need a system to tell us we need to know something.

In a trial of CME, a random sample of GPs were asked to rank 18 selected conditions into either a 'high preference' set, for which they wanted to receive CME or a 'low preference' set for which they did not want further education. Physicians with similar rankings were paired and randomised to either:

- a control group whose CME was postponed for 18 months; or

- an experimental group who received CME at once for their high preference topics and were also provided with training materials for their low preference topics and asked to promise to study them.

The outcomes were measured in terms of the quality of clinical care (QOC) provided by each of the physicians before and after CME (determined from clinical records). The results showed that although the knowledge of experimental physicians rose after their CME, the effects on QOC were disappointing with a similar (small) increase in QOC for both the experimental and control groups for their high preference conditions.

By contrast, for low preference conditions, QOC rose significantly for the experimental physicians but fell for the control group.

A review of didactic CME by Davies et al (1999) also concluded that formal sessions are not effective in changing physician performance (see Part 3: Resources and further reading).

Conclusions of CME trial

1. When you want CME, you don't need it.

2. CME only works when you don't want it.

3. CME does not cause general improvements in the quality of care.

Reference:

Sibley JC, Sackett DL, Neufeld V et al (1982). A randomised trial of continuing medical education. New England Journal of Medicine 306:511–515.

Overall, as we have seen, there is too much information but we still need it. The quality of most of the information is also very poor: most published information is irrelevant and/or the methods are not good. Finding the high-quality evidence is like trying to sip pure water from a water hose pumping dirty water, or looking for 'rare pearls'.

High quality/relevant data — pearls

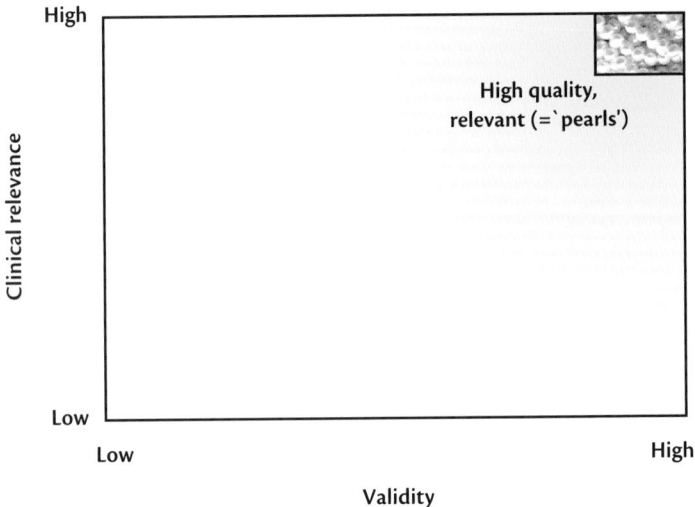

How many questions can doctors answer each day?

Many questions arise every day as a result of seeing people in clinical practice. Two papers have been published about this: one of interns in a hospital setting and one of GPs. In both cases, the researchers asked the doctors to note every time a question arose and what information they needed.

The study of 100 GPs showed that they each wrote down about 10 questions over a two and a half day period. The GPs tried to find answers for about half of these. The most critical factor influencing which questions they followed up was how long they thought it would take to get an answer. If the doctor thought the answer would be available in less than a couple of minutes, they were prepared to look for it. If they thought it would take longer, they would not bother. Only two questions in the whole study (ie 2/1000) were followed up using a proper electronic search.

Doctors' information needs

Study 1 (interns)

- 64 residents in 2 hospitals were interviewed after 401 consultations
- They asked an average of 280 questions (2 per 3 patients)
- Pursued an answer for 80 questions (29%)
- Others not pursued because of:
  - lack of time, or
  - because they forgot the question
- Souces of answers:
  - textbooks (31%)
  - articles (21%)
  - consultants (17%)

Study 2 (GPs)

- 103 GPs in Iowa collected questions over 2.5 days
- A total of 1101 questions were collected
- Pursued answers for 702 questions (64%)
- Spent less than 2 minutes pursuing an answer using readily available print and human resources
- Only 2 questions (0.2%) led to a formal literature search

References:

Green ML, Ciampi MA and Ellis PJ (2000). Residents' medical information needs in clinic: are they being met? American Journal of Medicine 109: 218–233.

Ely JW, Osheroff JA, Ebell MH et al (1999). Analysis of questions asked by family doctors regarding patient care. British Medical Journal 319:358–361.

Information gathering

There are two ways in which we all get information: 'push' and 'pull'.

'Push' new relevant and valid results

The 'push' method of getting our information is when we extract information from the variety of sources that we receive, across a wide spectrum of topics that may interest us. This is sometimes called 'just in case' learning.

For EBM, the best sources for the 'push' approach to improving knowledge are where the 'pearls' have already been selected from the rest of the lower quality literature. Some good sources of information where this has been done include:

Evidence-Based Medicine — a journal containing information from clinicians around the world who spot articles that pass rigorous validity criteria and are important to clinical practice. The journal is published every two months and has no original articles but it gives a condensed version of the original paper.

Also available on the internet at: **http://www.evidence-basedmedicine.com**

Clinical Evidence — is a compendium of evidence based literature searches. It is updated and published every six months as a book and CD. It is arranged by specialty and just states the best existing evidence for an intervention. If there is no evidence, it says so. It does not include opinions or consensus guidelines. The editors decide what questions are relevant but the book is based on what doctors need. Doctors can look up information when they need it (the 'pull' method of obtaining information).

Clinical Evidence is available on the internet at:
http://www.clinicalevidence.com

'Pull' answers in less then two minutes

In this workbook we focus on how to formulate questions and 'pull' answers out of the literature in less than two minutes! This is sometimes called 'just in time' learning. In the next sections we will look at some case studies where EBM methods were used and then find out how to frame a question to make it easier to answer. Then we will learn about how to use MEDLINE and the Cochrane databases to electronically search for the information we need and, finally, how to use the results.

Balance your information: 'pull' and 'push'

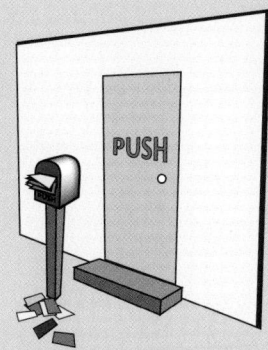

'Push' is when we receive information from a variety of sources and on a variety of topics and extract what we think we need for our practice ('just in case' learning).

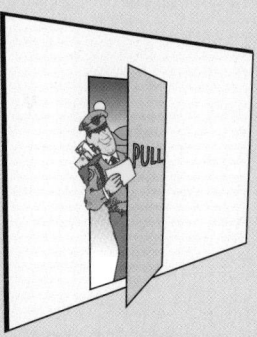

'Pull' is when we deliberately seek information to answer a specific question ('just in time' learning).

Some evidence-based cases

In this session, we will discuss several case studies that show how EBM can help in a range of clinical situations. You can then think of your own clinical question which you would like to answer at the workshop.

Case study 1: persistent cough

A 58-year-old who was visiting her GP about another matter, said, as an aside: 'Can you do anything about a cough?' She had had a persistent cough for 20 years with various treatments but no cure. She had been referred twice to physicians.

The GP searched PubMed (the web-based version of MEDLINE) using 'Clinical Queries', which is a category of PubMed designed for clinicians (see pages 52–54). The search for persistent cough revealed that the most common causes of a persistent cough are:

- postnasal drip
- asthma
- chronic bronchitis

The GP thought the cough was most likely to be due to asthma, and prescribed appropriate treatment for asthma as a first line of treatment. The patient thought she had already tried that treatment and that it did not work but tried it again anyway, without success. However, the search also showed that gastro-oesophageal reflux is a less common but possible cause of persistent cough (10% of cases), which the GP had not known before. The GP therefore recommended the patient to take antacids at night and raise the head of her bed. After one week her cough disappeared for the first time in 20 years and has not come back since.

How did EBM help?

This case raises interesting questions of what doctors 'should' know. It was written up in the British Medical Journal and published as an example of how EBM can help GPs. However, some physicians wrote in saying that 'everyone should know' that gastro-oesophageal reflux was a possible cause of cough. The author replied that although respiratory physicians might know this information, GPs did not necessarily know it. An anaesthetist wrote in to say that after reading the article he had been treated for gastro-oesophageal reflux, which had cured a cough he had had for 30 years!

Conclusion: EBM can help you find the information you need, whether or not you 'should' already know it.

Reference:

Glasziou P (1998). Evidence based case report: Twenty year cough in a non-smoker. British Medical Journal 316:1660–1661.

Case study 2: dog bite

A person came to the clinic with a fresh dog bite. It looked clean and the GP and patient wondered whether it was necessary to give prophylactic antibiotics. She searched MEDLINE and found a meta-analysis indicating that the average infection rate for dog bites was 14% and that antibiotics halved this risk. In other words:

- for every 100 people with dog bites, treatment with antibiotics will save 7 from getting infected; or

- treating 14 people with dog bites will prevent one infection.

The second number (14) is called the 'number needed to treat' (NNT).

The GP explained these figures to the patient, along with the possible consequences of an infection, and the patient decided not to take antibiotics. On follow-up it was found that the patient did not get infected.

How did EBM help?

In this case EBM helped because the empirical data were easy for the patient to understand and she could participate in the clinical decision. As the culture of health care changes further towards consumer participation in health care decision making, patients will demand this type of information.

Reference:

Cummings P (1994). Antibiotics to prevent infection in patients with dog bite wounds: a meta-analysis of randomized trials. Annals of Emergency Medicine 23:535–540.

Empirical measures of outcomes

Outcomes are commonly measured as absolute risk reduction (ARR), relative risks (RR) and number needed to treat (NNT).

The risk of infection after dog bite with no antibiotics
$$= 14\% \ (0.14)$$

The risk of infection after dog bite with antibiotics
$$= 7\% \ (0.07)$$

The ARR for antibiotic treatment
$$= 14 - 7 = 7\%$$
(That is, 7 people in every 100 treated will be saved from infection.)

$$NNT = 100/7$$
$$= 14$$
(That is, you would need to treat 14 dog bite patients with antibiotics to prevent 1 infection.)

RR of infection with antibiotics compared to without antibiotics
$$= 0.07/0.14$$
$$= 0.5 \ (50\%)$$

NOTE : It is best to quote the ARR or NNT in discussions with patients. RR is harder to put into context because it is independent of the frequency of the problem (the 'event rate'), in this case, the rate at which people with dog bites get infected. Further information on these measures is given in EBM Step 4 (Rapid critical appraisal).

Case study 3: microscopic blood in the urine

One of us, then a healthy 47-year-old male, was acting as a patient in a medical exam. The students accurately found microscopic traces of blood in his urine when they tested it. He went to his GP and was retested a month later. The blood was still there. The GP suggested conventional investigation: an ultrasound and cystoscopy. It was time for a search of the literature for evidence of the effectiveness of these procedures.

He searched for a cohort study of 40–50-year-olds with haematuria with long-term follow-up and for RCTs of screening for haematuria. He used the search categories 'prognosis' and 'specificity' and the search terms 'haematuria OR hematuria'. He got 300 hits. Two papers were very relevant (see box).

The presenter concluded that blood in urine is not a good indicator of bladder cancer and did not have the cystoscopy test.

How did EBM help?

The lesson from this case concerns the practical versus the empirical. Doctors tend to think along the lines of:

> Blood does not belong in the urine so it must be coming from somewhere. It could be coming from a potentially serious cause, such as bladder cancer.

Empirical questions, on the other hand, ask about outcomes — in this case whether conventional investigation leads to better health outcomes. In this case, the evidence (surprisingly) showed no benefit from this, because microscopic haematuria seems to be no more prevalent among those who later develop urological cancer than those who do not. Once again, this allows patients to participate much more fully in clinical decisions.

EBM can also help reduce litigation

This case raises the issue of possible litigation. What if the patient is not tested and later develops a serious disease? However, because EBM improves communication between doctors and patients and allows patients to share decision making, it protects doctors from litigation (most litigation happens when there is a breakdown in communication). EBM analyses have already been used in the courts and have been well accepted. Such empirical evidence has saved doctors from trouble when opinion may have damned them.

Study 1

10,000 men were screened. About 250 (2.5%) had haematuria. These men were asked to visit their GP and about 150 (60%) did so. Of those, only three had a serious problem. Of these:

- 2 had bladder cancer
- 1 had reflux nephropathy.

This shows that there is about a 1 in 50 chance of having a serious disease.

Study 2

A urine test to 20,000 men as part of a work-based personal health appraisal. Follow-up studies of the men who were positive for haematuria found three cancers per year, or 1.5 cancers per 1000 person-years. However, the people who were not found to have haematuria were also followed up and the rate of cancer was exactly the same as for the people with haematuria.

Reference:

Del Mar C (2000). Asymptomatic haematuria … in the doctor. British Medical Journal 320:165–166.

Case study 4: painful shoulder

A 68-year-old male complained of a painful left shoulder for several weeks. His GP had often used cortisone injections for such shoulder pain, but was now not sure if this was a good idea because she had seen a recent trial of cortisone injection for tennis elbow which showed good short-term improvement but the long-term outcomes were worse than with watchful-waiting or physiotherapy. A search of the Cochrane Library found a systematic review of randomised trials of several treatments for shoulder pain, which was last updated in 1999.

Based on two small trials (with a total of 90 patients), the authors concluded that subacromial steroid injection showed some short-term benefit over placebo. A further search of the Clinical Trials Registry identified a more recent trial that compared physiotherapy, manipulation and corticosteroid injections in a total of 172 patients. It showed that corticosteroid injections had short-term benefits (up to 1 year) with a 50% absolute increase in 'cure' at 11 weeks. However, when long-term outcomes were measured (2–3 years), about half the patients had some recurrence and there was no difference between the three groups.

How did EBM help?

The search revealed studies that answered the GP's question and provided useful information for the patient. The GP was able to advise her patient of three things:

- he would probably improve even without treatment

- a steroid injection would help to relieve pain in the short-term (up to 1 year)

- a steroid injection would make no difference in the long term (2–3 years).

Based on this information, the patient was able to make an informed decision about whether to have the injection or not.

References:

Green S, Buchbinder R, Glazier R, Forbes A (2002). Interventions for shoulder pain (Cochrane Review). In: The Cochrane Library, Issue 2, 2002. Oxford: Update Software.

Winters JC, Jorritsma W, Groenier KH et al (1999). Treatment of shoulder complaints in general practice: long term results of a randomised, single blind study comparing physiotherapy, manipulation, and corticosteroid injection. British Medical Journal 318:1395–1396.

Summary of case studies

The case studies show that EBM has several advantages:

- Medical practitioners, especially GPs, can't know everything. EBM helps doctors keep up to date across a very wide spectrum of information.

- MEDLINE and similar databases have several advantages. For medical practitioners, they are a way of finding up-to-date information that is not biased and is of good quality.

- Because the search is based on questions rather than possible answers, doctors can find information without having heard about it before. In other words, they can find information that they do not initially know they need, but which, as we have seen, is important for good clinical practice.

- The evidence can be used to quantify outcomes (empirical evidence). It allows people to assess the likelihood of benefiting from a particular treatment or activity rather than just considering the underlying mechanism.

- Patients like this empirical approach because it is easier to understand and allows them to share in decision making.

- Decision making can be shared between the doctor and patient based on empirical evidence of risks and benefits. This reduces the chances of future litigation.

- Electronic searching can reveal other useful information that is of benefit to the patient.

Participants' own clinical questions

Now we will work out how to turn your day-to-day questions into structured questions that can be answered in a similar way to the case studies above.

In the space provided below, write down a question in relation to either yourself or one of your patients. If you are stuck, write down the last patient you saw and we will work out a question.

In the next section (page 23), we will look at how to turn your questions into a form that can be used to search the medical literature in less than two minutes. Then we will use the computer lab to find answers to them.

Write down a clinical question here

Notes

Part 2

The steps in evidence-based medicine

EBM

EBM step 1: Formulate an answerable question

First principle

First, you must admit that you don't know.

As we have already seen, it is impossible to know everything. EBM gives you a method to find answers to questions without having any prior knowledge of what you ought to know.

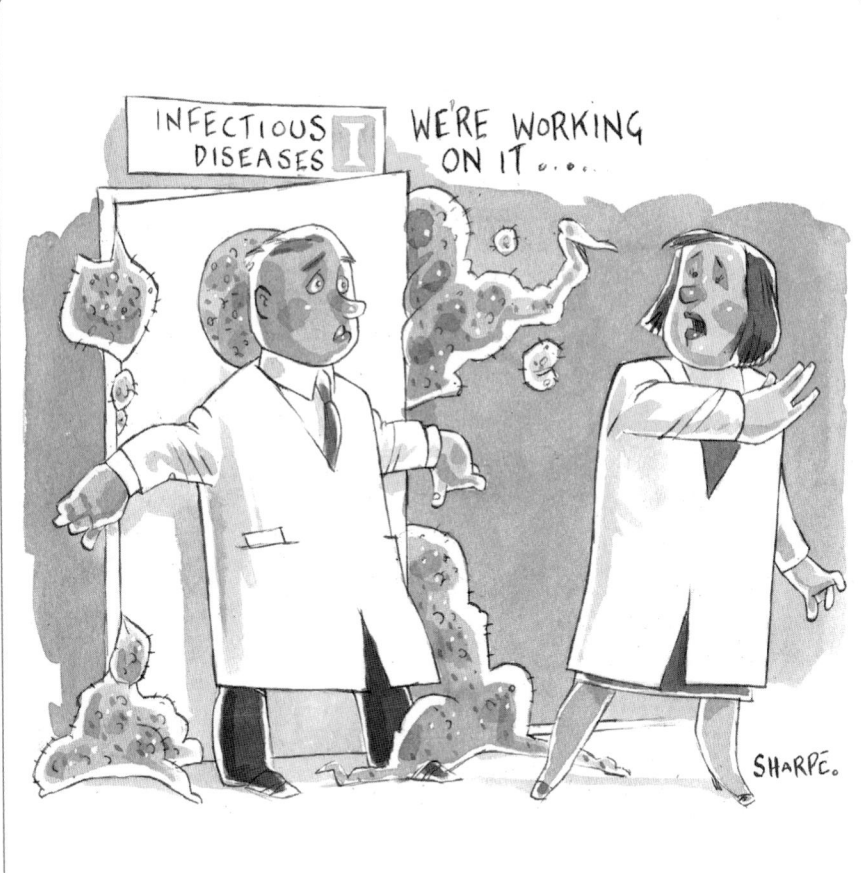

Steps in EBM:

1. Formulate an answerable question.

2. Track down the best evidence of outcomes available.

3. Critically appraise the evidence (ie find out how good it is).

4. Apply the evidence (integrate the results with clinical expertise and patient values).

5. Evaluate the effectiveness and efficiency of the process (to improve next time).

The 'PICO' principle

Questions often spring to mind in a form that makes finding answers in the medical literature a challenge. Dissecting the question into its component parts and restructuring it so that it is easy to find the answers is an essential first step in EBM. Most questions can be divided into 4 parts:

1. The **population or participants**	Who are the relevant patients?
2. The **intervention or indicator**	What is the management strategy, diagnostic test or exposure that you are interested in (such as a drug, food, surgical procedure, diagnostic test or exposure to a chemical)?
3. The **comparator or control**	What is the control or alternative management strategy, test or exposure that you will be comparing the one you are interested in with?
4. The **outcome**	What are the patient-relevant consequences of the exposure in which we are interested?

All clinical or research questions can be divided into these four components, which we call 'P I C O'. It is important to use all four parts of the question, if possible.

Remember the PICO principle

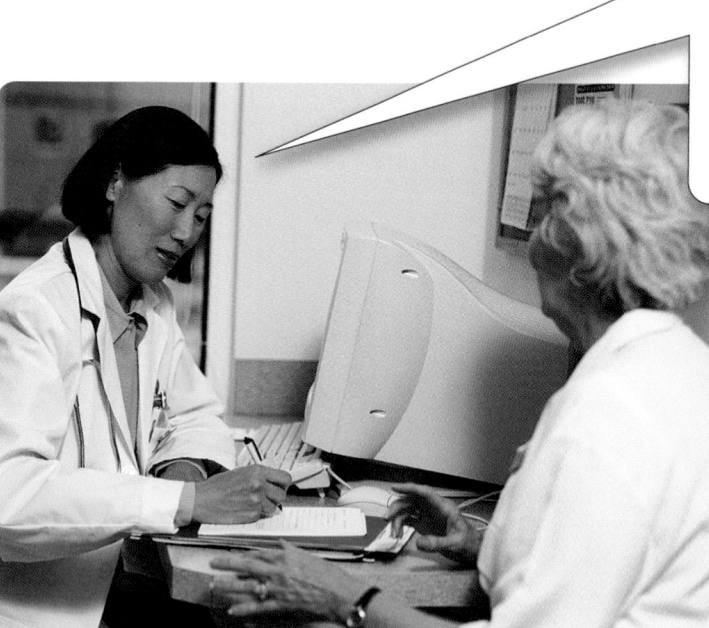

P Population/patient

I Intervention/indicator

C Comparator/control

O Outcome

Different types of questions

By far the most common type of clinical question is about how to treat a disease or condition. In EBM, treatments and therapies are called 'interventions' and such questions are questions of INTERVENTION.

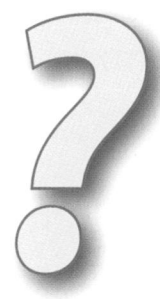

However, not all research questions are about interventions. Other types of questions that may arise are as follows:

1. What causes the problem? AETIOLOGY AND RISK FACTORS

2. What is the frequency of the problem? FREQUENCY

3. Does this person have the problem? DIAGNOSIS

4. Who will get the problem? PROGNOSIS AND PREDICTION

In each case the P I C O method can be used to formulate the question, as shown in the following examples. The same approach can be used to research qualitative questions about health issues of a more general nature (PHENOMENA). In this case, the question will consist of 'P' and 'O' only.

The studies that you will need to search for are different for the different types of questions and we will discuss this further in the next section (see 'EBM step 2: Track down the best evidence').

Interventions

Interventions cover a wide range of activities from drug treatments and other clinical therapies, to lifestyle changes (for example, diet or exercise) and social activities (such as an education program). Interventions can include individual patient care or population health activities (for example, screening for diseases such as cervical or prostate cancer).

Example 1

A 28-year-old male presents with recurrent furunculosis for past 8 months; these episodes have been treated with drainage and several courses of antibiotics but keep recurring. He asks if recurrences can be prevented.

To convert this to an answerable question, use the P I C O method as follows :

P *Population/patient* = patients with recurrent furunculosis

I *Intervention/indicator* = prophylactic antibiotics

C *Comparator/control* = no treatment

O *Outcome* = reduction in recurrence rate of furunculosis

Question:

'In patients with recurrent furunculosis, do prophylactic antibiotics, compared to no treatment, reduce the recurrence rate?'

Example 2

Jeff, a smoker of more than 30 years, has come to see you about something unrelated. You ask him if he is interested in stopping smoking. He tells you he has tried to quit smoking unsuccessfully in the past. A friend of his, however, successfully quit with accupuncture. Should he try it? Other interventions you know about are nicotine replacement therapy and antidepressants.

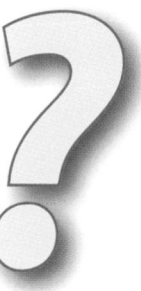

Develop a clinical research question using P I C O:

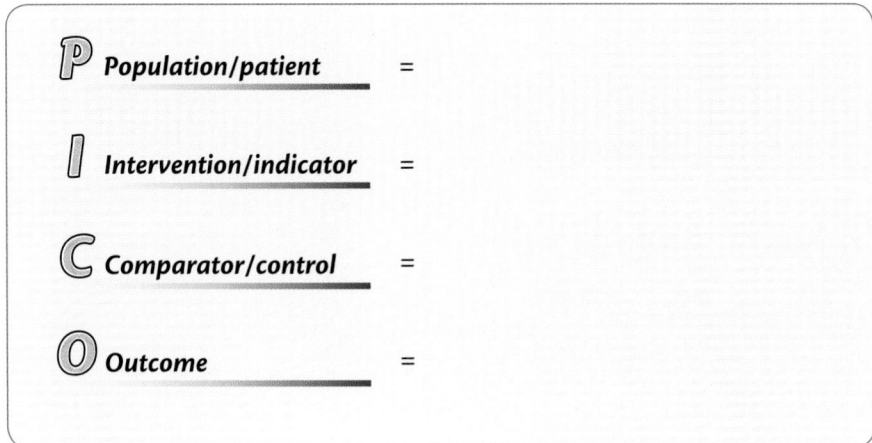

P Population/patient   =

I Intervention/indicator   =

C Comparator/control   =

O Outcome   =

Question:

Example 3

At a routine immunisation visit, Lisa, the mother of a 6-month-old, tells you that her baby suffered a nasty local reaction after her previous immunisation. Lisa is very concerned that the same thing may happen again this time. Recently, a colleague told you that needle length can affect local reactions to immunisation in young children but can't remember the precise details.

Develop a clinical research question using P I C O to help you find the information you need:

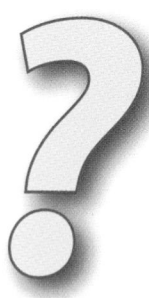

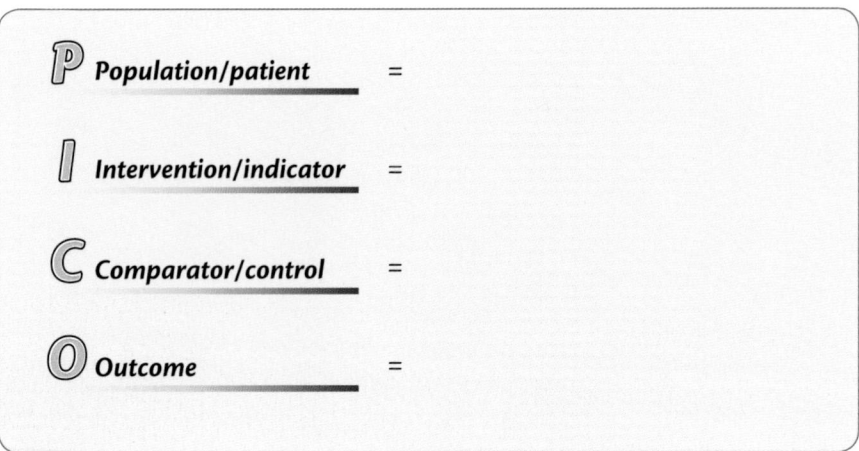

P **Population/patient**   =

I **Intervention/indicator**   =

C **Comparator/control**   =

O **Outcome**   =

Question:

Example 4

In browsing one of the medical weeklies, you come across mention of imiquimod cream for treatment of basal cell carcinomas (BCC). The idea of a cream for BCCs is surprising, so you wonder about the effectiveness and particularly the long-term cure rate of imiquimod cream.

Develop a clinical research question using P I C O to help answer your query:

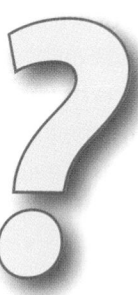

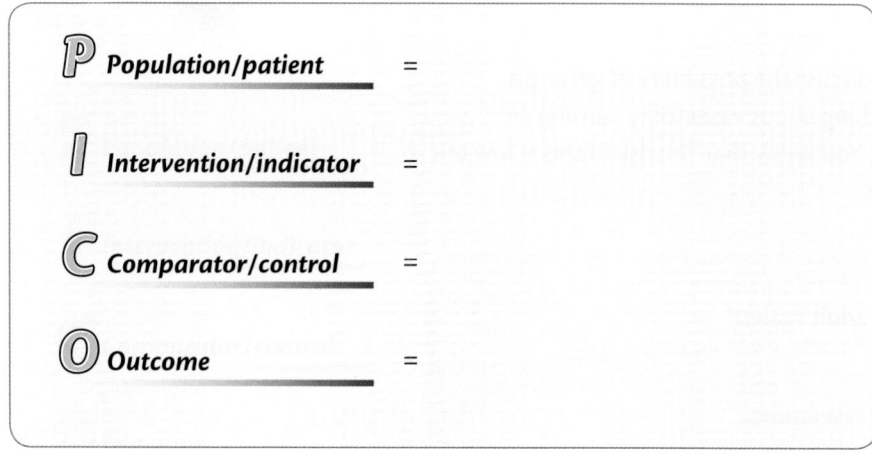

P **Population/patient** =

I **Intervention/indicator** =

C **Comparator/control** =

O **Outcome** =

Question:

Frequency or rate

Questions of *frequency* (prevalence) are about how many people in the population have a disease or health problem, such as what is the frequency of hearing problems in infants or the prevalence of Alzheimer's disease in the over 70s. If the question also includes a time period, such as for cases of influenza in winter versus summer, it becomes a question of *rate* (incidence).

Example 1

Mabel is a 6-week-old baby at her routine follow-up. She was born prematurely at 35 weeks. You want to tell the parents about her chances of developing hearing problems.

P **Population/patient** = infants

I **Intervention/indicator** = premature

C **Comparator/control** = full-term

O **Outcome** = sensorial deafness

Question:

'In infants born prematurely, compared to those born at full term, what will the prevalence of sensorial deafness be?'

Example 2

Mrs Smith has acute lower back pain. She has never had such pain before and is convinced that it must be caused by something really serious. You take a history and examine her but find no indicators of a more serious condition. You reassure her that the majority of acute low back pain is not serious but she is still not convinced.

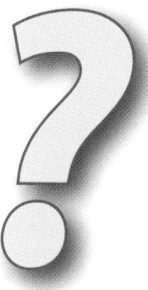

Develop a clinical research question using P I C O to help reassure Mrs Smith:

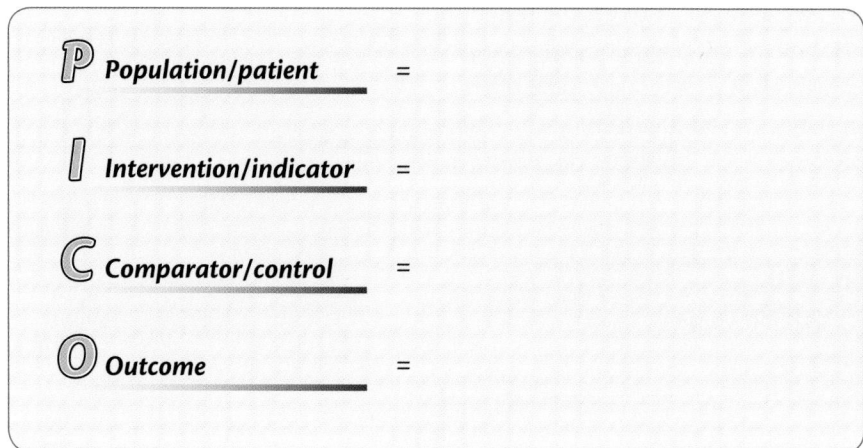

P *Population/patient* =

I *Intervention/indicator* =

C *Comparator/control* =

O *Outcome* =

Question:

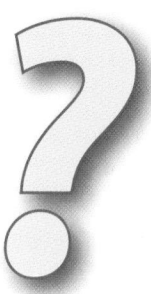

Diagnosis

Diagnosis questions are concerned with how accurate a diagnostic test is in various patient groups and in comparison to other available tests. Measures of test accuracy include its sensitivity and specificity.

Example 1

Julie is pregnant for the second time. She had her first baby when she was 33 and had amniocentesis to find out if the baby had Down syndrome. The test was negative but it was not a good experience as she did not get the result until she was 18 weeks pregnant. She is now 35, one month pregnant and asks if she can have a test that would give her an earlier result. The local hospital offers serum biochemistry plus nuchal translucency ultrasound screening as a first trimester test for Down syndrome. You wonder if this combination of tests is as reliable as conventional amniocentesis.

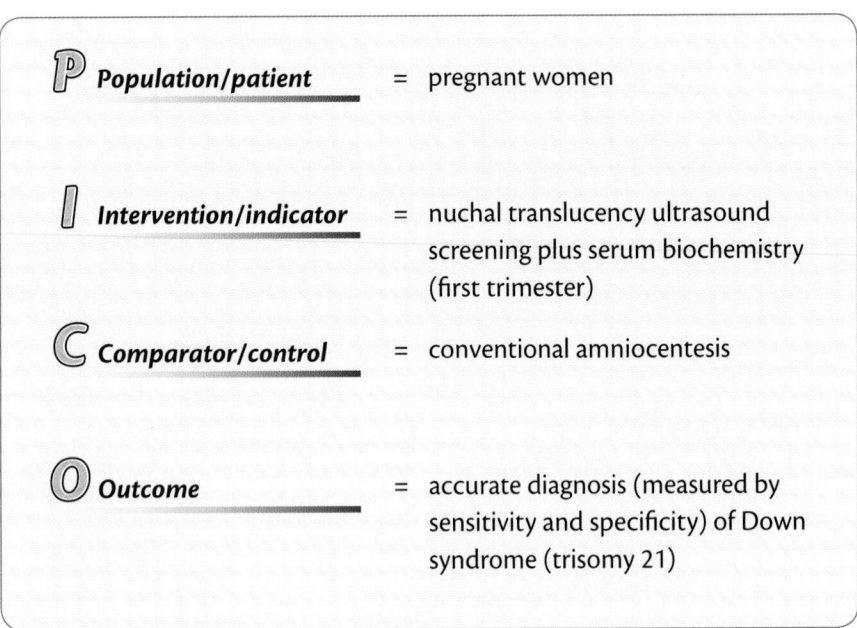

P Population/patient	=	pregnant women
I Intervention/indicator	=	nuchal translucency ultrasound screening plus serum biochemistry (first trimester)
C Comparator/control	=	conventional amniocentesis
O Outcome	=	accurate diagnosis (measured by sensitivity and specificity) of Down syndrome (trisomy 21)

Question:

'For pregnant women, is nuchal translucency ultrasound screening plus serum biochemistry testing in the first trimester as accurate (ie with equal or better sensitivity and specificity) as conventional amniocentesis for diagnosing Down syndrome?'

Example 2

As part of your clinic's assessment of elderly patients, there is a check of hearing. Over a tea room discussion it turns out that some people simply ask and others use a tuning fork, but you claim that a simple whispered voice test is very accurate. Challenged to back this up with evidence, you promise to do a literature search before tomorrow's meeting.

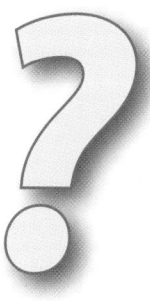

Develop a clinical research question using P I C O to help you with your literature research:

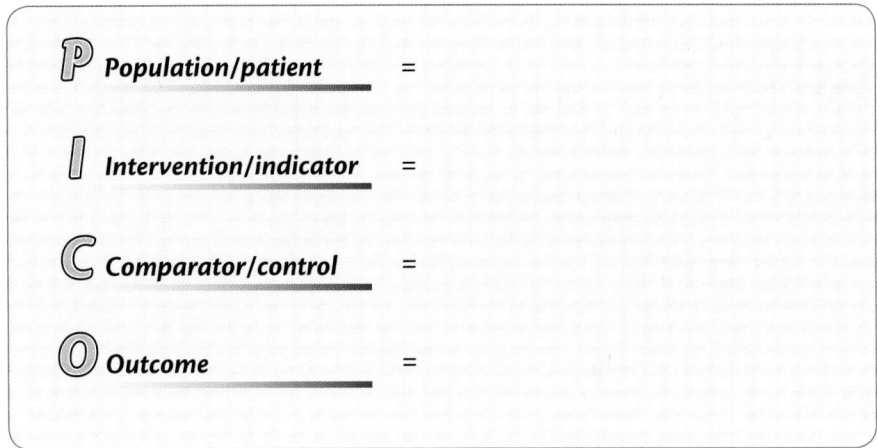

P **Population/patient** =

I **Intervention/indicator** =

C **Comparator/control** =

O **Outcome** =

Question:

Prediction (prognosis)

Prediction or prognosis questions are concerned with how likely an outcome is for a population with certain characteristics (risk factors), such as the likelihood that a man who is experiencing atypical chest pains will suffer further heart failure or sudden death within the next few days, or the predicted morbidity and mortality for a person diagnosed with colon cancer.

Example 1

Childhood seizures are common and frightening for the parents and the decision to initiate prophylactic treatment after a first fit is a difficult one. To help parents make their decision, you need to explain the risk of further occurrences following a single seizure of unknown cause.

P Population/patient	=	children
I Intervention/indicator	=	one seizure of unknown cause
C Comparator/control	=	no seizures
O Outcome	=	further seizures

Question:

'In children who have had one seizure of unknown cause, compared with children who have had no seizures, what is the increased risk of further seizures?'

Example 2

Mr Thomas, who is 58 years old, has correctly diagnosed his inguinal lump as a hernia. He visits you for confirmation of his diagnosis and information about the consequences. You mention the possibility of strangulation, and the man asks: 'How likely is that?' You reply 'pretty unlikely' (which is as much as you know at the time) but say that you will try and find out more precisely.

Develop a clinical research question using P I C O to help you give Mr Thomas more precise details about his prognosis:

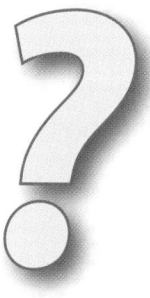

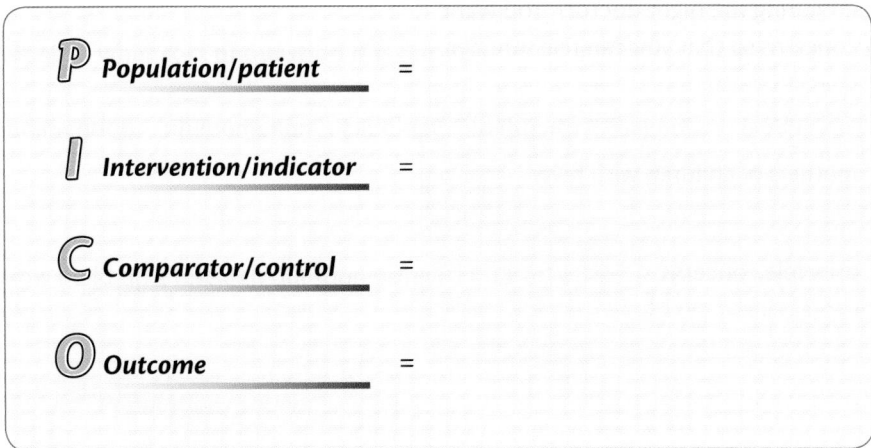

P *Population/patient* =

I *Intervention/indicator* =

C *Comparator/control* =

O *Outcome* =

Question:

Your own questions

2. Write a second clinical issue that interests you.

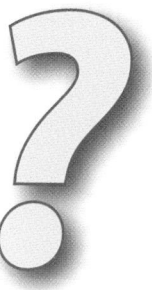

Identify what sort of question it is (circle):

intervention   phenomenon   aetiology   frequency   diagnosis   prediction

Now build up a research question using P I C O

P Population/patient	=
I Intervention/indicator	=
C Comparator/control	=
O Outcome	=

Question:

Types of studies

The types of studies that give the best evidence are different for the different types of questions. In every case, however, the best evidence comes from studies where the methods used maximise the chance of eliminating bias. The study designs that best suit the different question types outlined are as follows:

Question	Best study designs	Description
INTERVENTION	Randomised controlled trial	Subjects are randomly allocated to treatment or control groups and outcomes assessed.
AETIOLOGY AND RISK FACTORS	Randomised controlled trial	As aetiology questions are similar to intervention questions, the ideal study type is an RCT. However, it is usually not ethical or practical to conduct such a trial to assess harmful outcomes.
	Cohort study	Outcomes are compared for matched groups with and without exposure or risk factor (prospective study).
	Case-control study	Subjects with and without outcome of interest are compared for previous exposure or risk factor (retrospective study).
FREQUENCY AND RATE	Cohort study	As above
	Cross-sectional study	Measurement of condition in a representative (preferably random) sample of people.
DIAGNOSIS	Cross-sectional study with random or consecutive sample	Preferably an independent, blind, comparison with 'gold standard' test.
PROGNOSIS AND PREDICTION	Cohort /survival study	Long-term follow-up of a representative cohort.
PHENOMENA	Qualitative	Narrative analysis, or focus group; designed to assess the range of issues (rather than their quantification).

In each case, a systematic review of all the available studies is better than an individual study.

Notes

EBM step 2: Track down the best evidence

Where to search

The two main databases of information that we will use to search for evidence are:

PubMed

National Library of Medicine free internet MEDLINE database.

http://www.ncbi.nlm.nih.gov/entrez/query.fcgi

The 'Clinical Queries' section of PubMed is a question-focused interface with filters for identifying the more appropriate studies for questions of therapy, prognosis, diagnosis and aetiology.

The Cochrane Library

The Cochrane Library contains all the information collected by the Cochrane Collaboration. It contains the following databases:

The Cochrane Database of Systematic Reviews	Cochrane systematic reviews
The Cochrane Controlled Trials Register	Register of clinical trials that have been carried out or are in progress. The register contains over 300,000 controlled trials, which is the best single repository in the world.
The Database of Abstracts of Reviews of Effectiveness (DARE)	Structured abstracts of systematic reviews

Access to the Cochrane Library is free for users in many countries.

http://www.cochrane.org and follow the prompts

Other useful places to search are shown in the 'Resources and further reading' section of this workbook.

Steps in EBM:

1. Formulate an answerable question.

2. Track down the best evidence of outcomes available.

3. Critically appraise the evidence (ie find out how good it is).

4. Apply the evidence (integrate the results with clinical expertise and patient values).

5. Evaluate the effectiveness and efficiency of the process (to improve next time).

The question guides the search

In the previous section we discussed how to break down any type of clinical question into four components:

P *Population/patient*

I *Intervention/indicator*

C *Comparator/control*

O *Outcome*

You can now use these components to direct your search. It is also worth looking for synonyms for each component.

General structure of question

(Population OR synonym1 OR synonym2...) AND

(Intervention OR synonym1 OR synonym2...) AND

(Comparator OR synonym1 OR synonym2...) AND

(Outcome OR synonym1 OR synonym2...)

Example:

Question: In adults screened with faecal occult blood-testing, compared to no screening, is there a reduction in mortality from colorectal cancer?

Question part	Question term	Synonyms
Population/setting	Adult, human	–
Intervention or indicator	Screening, colorectal cancer	Screen, early detection, bowel cancer
Comparator	No screening	–
Outcome	Mortality	Death*, survival

* = wildcard symbol (finds words with the same stem)

The parts of the question can also be represented as a Venn diagram:

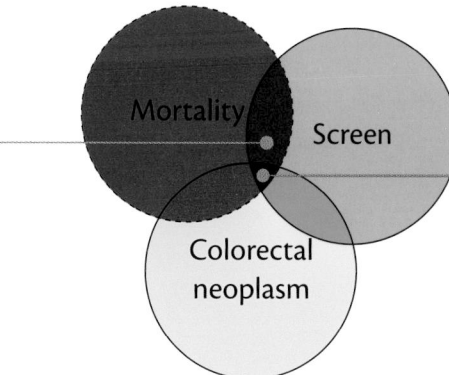

Once the study question has been broken down into its components, they can be combined using the Boolean operators 'AND' and 'OR'. For example:

> `(mortality AND screen)` — represents the overlap between these two terms — retrieves only articles that use both terms.
>
> `(screen AND colorectal neoplasm AND mortality)` — represents the small area where all three circles overlap — retrieves only articles with all three terms.

Complex combinations are possible. For example, the following combination captures all the overlap areas between the circles in the Venn diagram:

> `(mortality AND screen) OR (mortality AND colorectal neoplasms) OR (screen AND colorectal neoplasms)`

Although the overlap of all the parts of the question will generally have the best concentration of relevant articles, the other areas may still contain many relevant articles. Hence, if the disease AND study factor combination (solid circles in Venn diagram) is manageable, it is best to work with this and not further restrict by, for example, using outcomes (dotted circle in Venn diagram).

When the general structure of the question is developed it is worth looking for synonyms for each component.

Thus a search string might be:

> `(screen* OR early detection) AND (colorectal cancer OR bowel cancer) AND (mortality OR death* OR survival)`

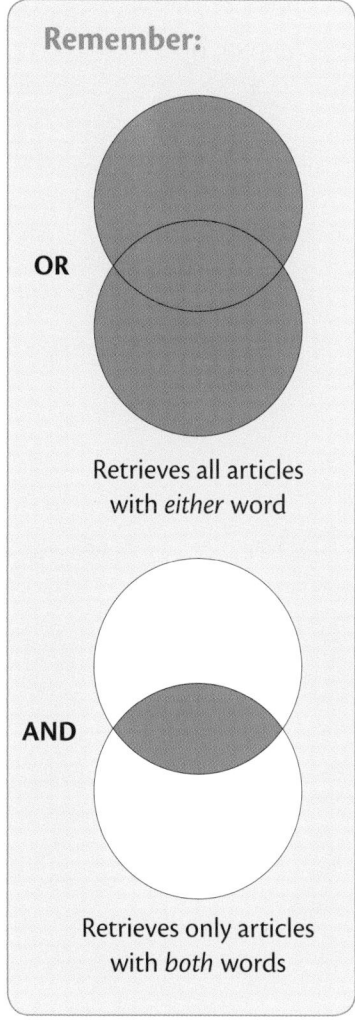

Remember:

OR

Retrieves all articles with *either* word

AND

Retrieves only articles with *both* words

The term 'screen*' is shorthand for words beginning with screen, for example, screen, screened, screening. (Note: the 'wildcard' symbol varies between systems, eg it may be an asterisk [*], or colon [:].)

In looking for synonyms you should consider both textwords and keywords in the database. The MEDLINE keyword system, known as MeSH (Medical Subject Heading), has a tree structure that covers a broad set of synonyms very quickly. The 'explode' (exp) feature of the tree structure allows you to capture an entire subtree of MeSH terms within a single word. Thus for the colorectal cancer term in the above search, the appropriate MeSH term might be:

```
colonic neoplasm (exp)
```

with the 'explode' incorporating all the MeSH tree below colonic neoplasm, viz:

```
colorectal neoplasms
        colonic polyps
                adenomatous polyposis coli
        colorectal neoplasms
                colorectal neoplasms, hereditary
                nonpolyposis
        sigmoid neoplasms
```

While the MeSH system is useful, it should supplement rather than replace the use of textwords so that incompletely coded articles are not missed.

The MeSH site can be accessed from PubMed (see 'How to use PubMed' later in this section).

Searching tips and tactics

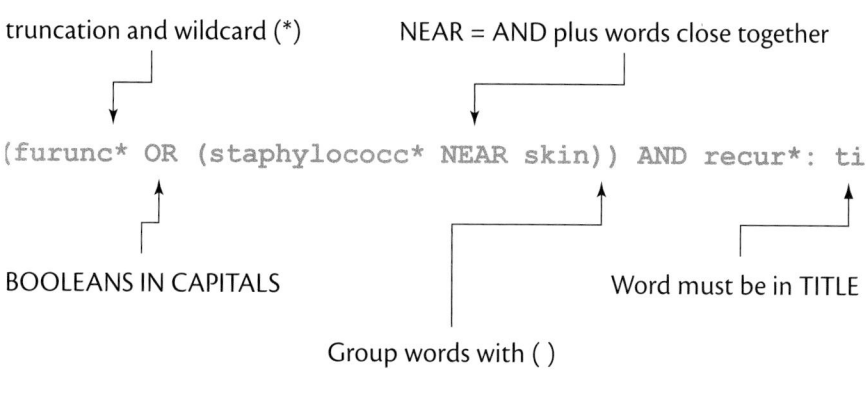

truncation and wildcard (*) NEAR = AND plus words close together

```
(furunc* OR (staphylococc* NEAR skin)) AND recur*: ti
```

BOOLEANS IN CAPITALS   Word must be in TITLE

Group words with ( )

OR	Finds studies containing either of the specified words or phrases. For example, `child OR adolescent` finds articles with either the word child or the word adolescent.
AND	Finds studies containing both specified words or phrases. For example, `child AND adolescent` finds articles with both the word child and the word adolescent.
NEAR	Like `AND`, `NEAR` requires both words but the specified words must also be within about 5 words from each other.
NOT	Excludes studies containing the specified word or phrase. For example, `child NOT adolescent` means studies with the word 'child' but not the word 'adolescent'. Use sparingly.
Limits	Articles retrieved may be restricted in several ways, eg by date, by language, by whether there is an abstract, etc.
()	Use parentheses to group words. For example, `(child OR adolescent) AND (hearing OR auditory)` finds articles with one or both 'child' and 'adolescent' and one or both of the words 'hearing' or 'auditory'.
*	Truncation: the '*'acts as a wildcard indicating any further letters, eg child* is child plus any further letters and is equivalent to `(child OR childs OR children OR childhood)`.
[ti] or:ti	Finds studies with the word in the title. For example, `hearing [ti]` (in PubMed) and `hearing:ti` (in Cochrane) finds studies with the word hearing in the title.
so or [so]	Retrieves studies from a specific source, eg `hearing AND BMJ [so]` finds articles on hearing in the BMJ.
MeSH	MeSH is the Medical Subject Headings, a controlled vocabulary of keywords which may be used in PubMed or Cochrane. It is often useful to use both MeSH heading and text words.

How to use the Cochrane Library

Go to the Cochrane Library homepage at:

http://www.cochrane.org and follow the prompts.

If you are in a registered country for use of the library you can use the 'Log on anonymously' button to log into the library.

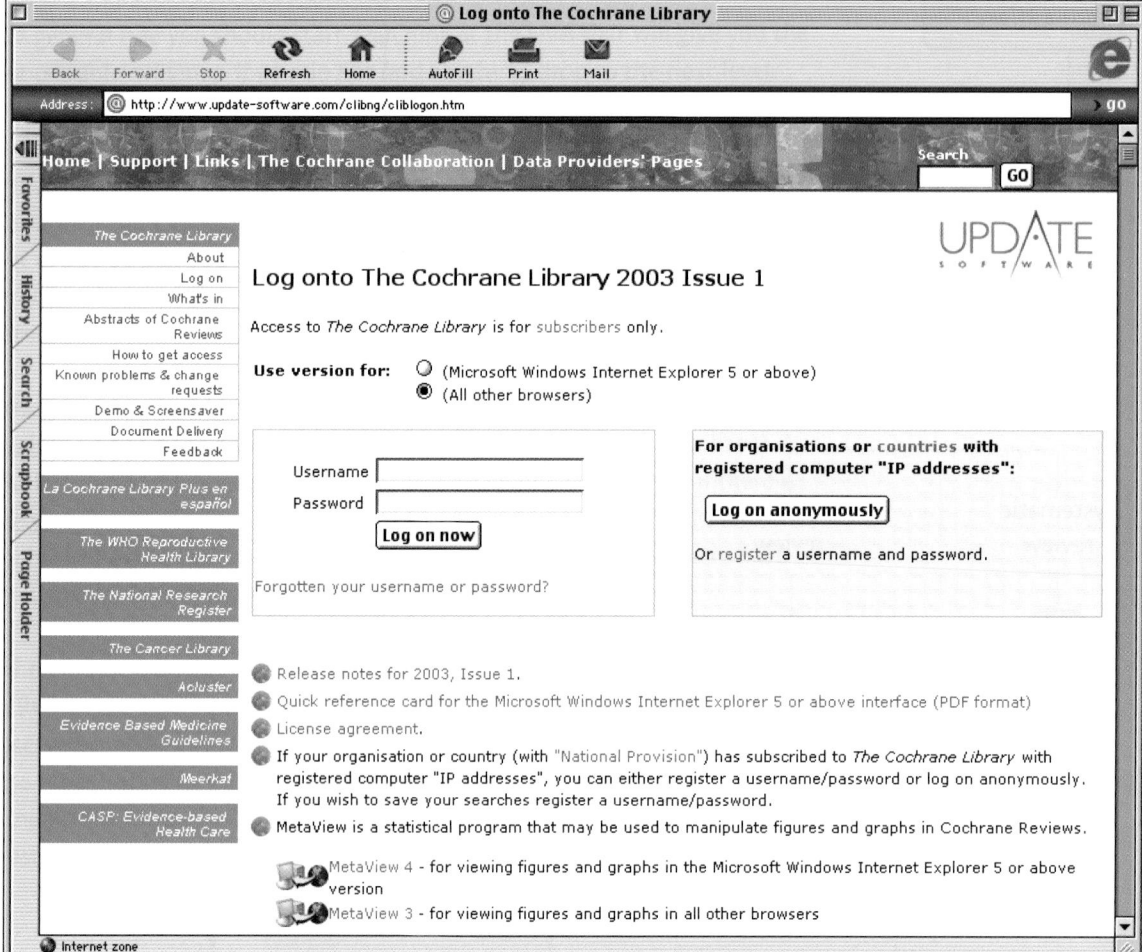

The library includes:

- The Cochrane Database of Systematic Reviews with approximately 1500 completed reviews and 1100 protocols (reviews that are currently in progress but not finished)

- Database of Abstracts of Reviews of Effectiveness (DARE) with about 3000 abstracts of other systematic reviews

- The Cochrane Central Register of Clinical Trials (CENTRAL), which lists over 350,000 controlled trials that have been carried out or are currently in progress, many with abstracts.

The screenshot on this page is reproduced with permission from update software

To search the library, enter your search phrase in the space provided. The results will show the total 'hits' from the site and the hits from each database. Click on each report to show the details.

Cochrane systematic reviews are very detailed but each has a structured abstract with the main findings. You can also go to the 'Tables and Graphs' section towards the end of the report and click on the studies to see the results of the analysis. These results can often be used to calculate a 'number needed to treat' (NNT).

For example, the search terms 'carpal tunnel AND corticosteroid' shows the following systematic review:

'Local corticosteroid treatment for carpal tunnel syndrome'

The 'Tables and Graphs' area of the review shows one study where corticosteroid treatment was compared to placebo treatment as the comparator with the numbers of patients showing improvement at 1 month as the outcome.

The results showed a statistically significant benefit at one month for the treated group of patients as follows:

	Number improved at 1 month	% improved
Hydrocortisone	23/30	77
Placebo	6/30	20
Percentage improved because of treatment		57 (57 better from 100 treated)
NNT		100/57 = 1.75 (ie more than 1 in every 2 patients treated will improve)

(Note: Symptom improvement beyond 1 month has not been demonstrated)

How to use PubMed

Go the the 'Entrez-PubMed' webpage at:

http://www.ncbi.nlm.nih.gov/entrez/query.fcgi

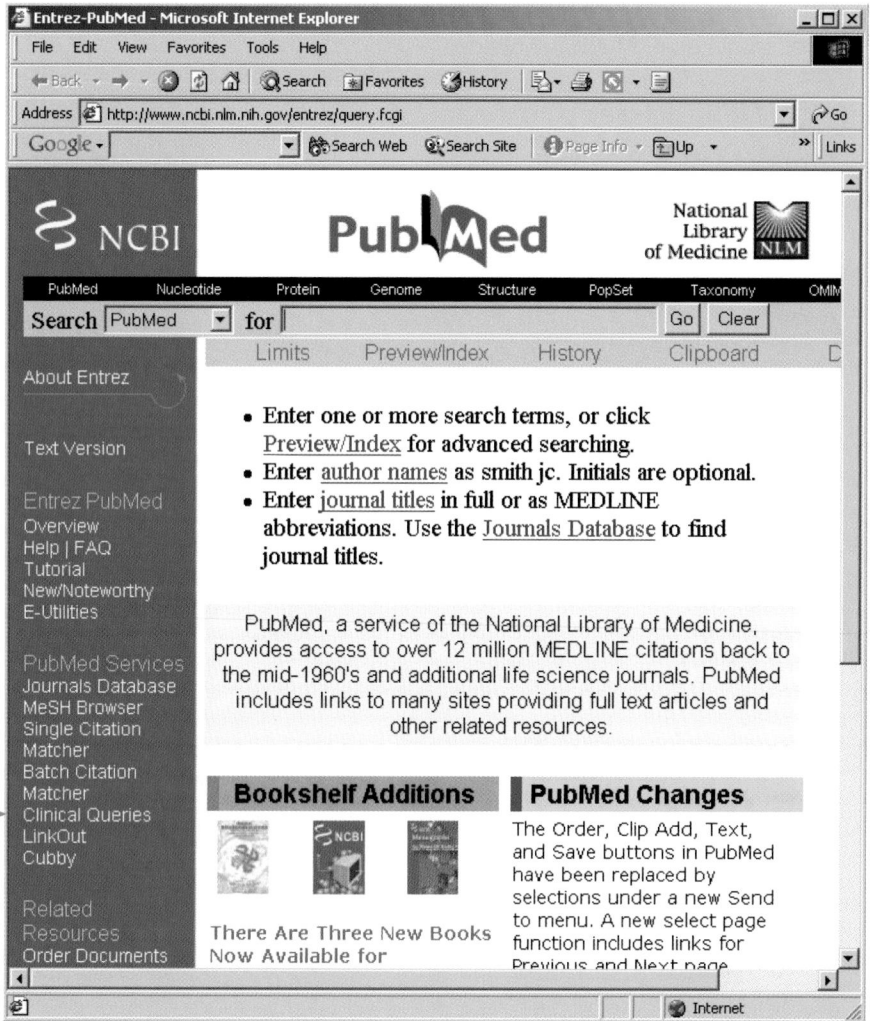

You can search directly from the entry page by typing your search terms into the box at the top. Click 'Limits' to set limits such as date, language and type of article. However, this sort of search does not provide any filtering for quality of the research and you will probably retrieve a large number of articles of variable usefulness.

To improve the quality of the studies you retrieve, click on 'Clinical Queries' on the sidebar.

The screenshots on p 52–3 are reproduced with permission. Source: The National Center for Biotechnology Information, The National Library of Medicine, The National Institute of Health, Department of Health and Human Services

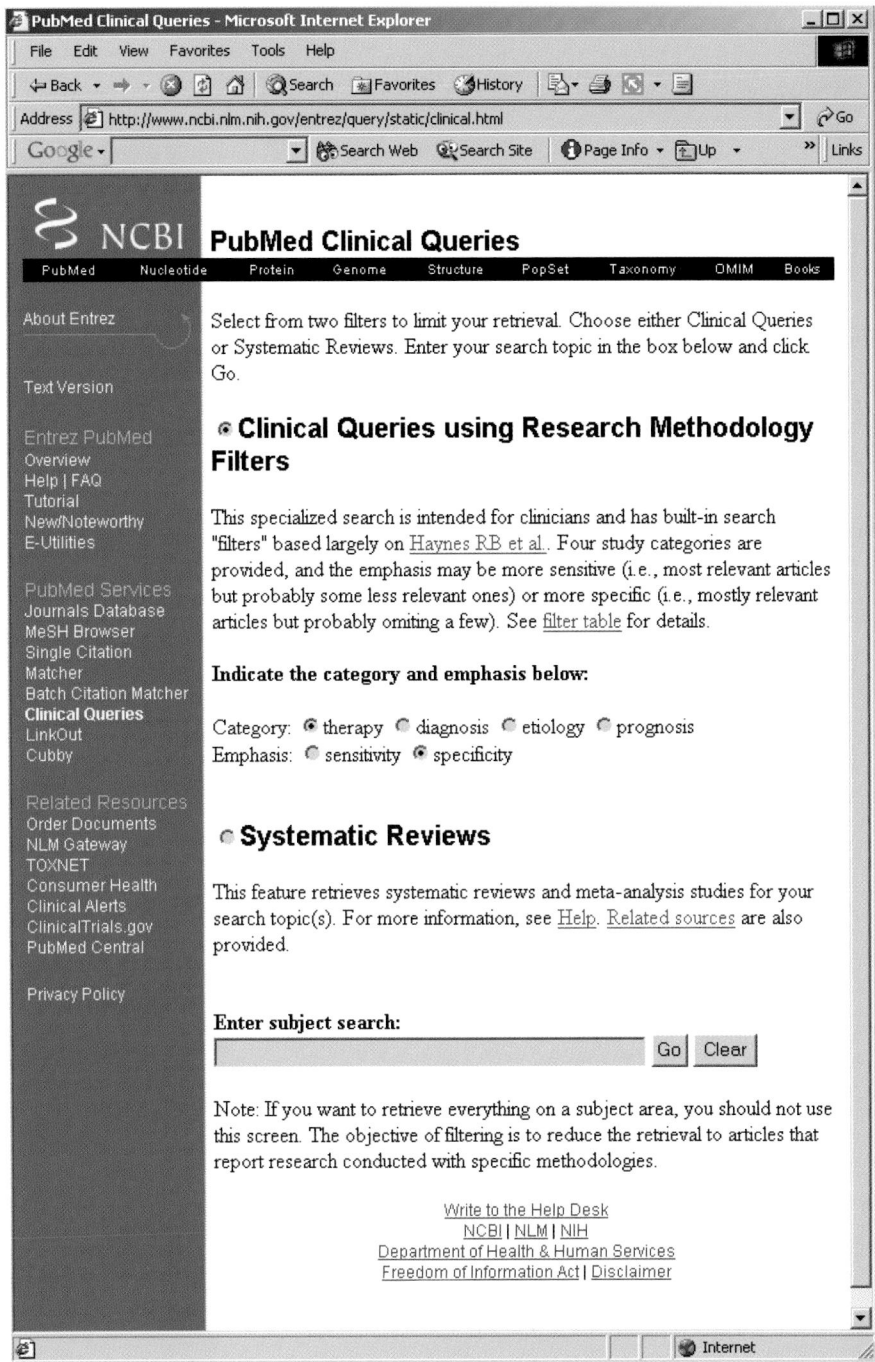

Next, enter the type of question you are trying to answer (ie intervention [therapy], diagnosis, aetiology, prognosis). If you click the 'Sensitivity' button you will get more articles but some may be less relevant. 'Specificity' gives you only highly relevant articles.

Finally, enter your search terms in the box and click 'Go'.

More about MeSH headings

From the PubMed entry page, click 'MeSH Browser' from the sidebar. In the next screen click 'MeSH'.

Next, click 'Online searching' to enter the search browser. Now you can enter the term you are looking for to get the full MeSH subject heading list for that topic.

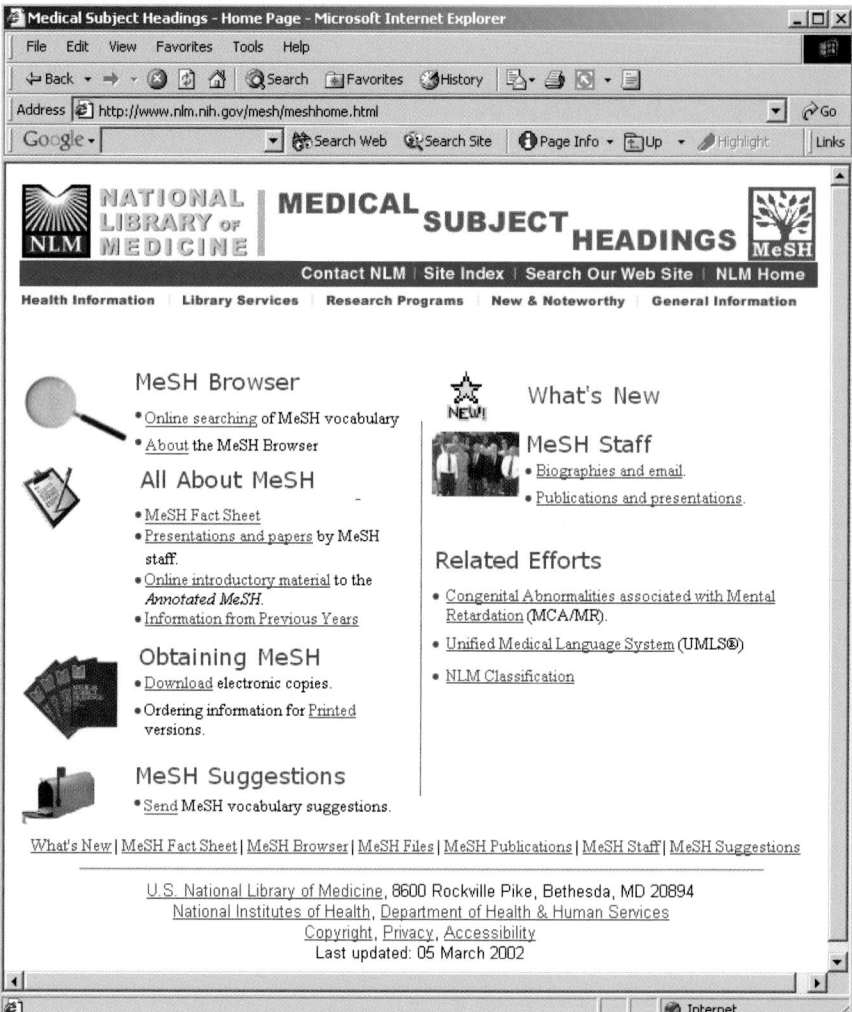

PubMed tutorial

PubMed has a detailed tutorial program. Click on 'Tutorial' on the side bar of the PubMed entry page. The tutorial is quite detailed and takes about 2 hours to go right through but it is very helpful.

Your search terms

Based on your 'P I C O' and question, write down some search terms and synonyms that you can use for your search:

Question 1:		

Question part	Question term	Synonyms
P **Population/patient**	(OR	)AND
I **Intervention/indicator**	(OR	)AND
C **Comparator/control**	(OR	)AND
O **Outcome**	(OR	)

Results of search

Remember to consider truncating words and using the * wildcard symbol, for example: *child** rather than *children*.

Question 2:		

Question part	Question term	Synonyms
P **Population/patient**	(OR	)AND
I **Intervention/indicator**	(OR	)AND
C **Comparator/control**	(OR	)AND
O **Outcome**	(OR	)

Results of search

Results

Question 1:

Cochrane Library search terms used:	Hits
Key references:	
Results (including absolute risk, NNT, etc if possible):	
PubMed search terms used:	Hits
Key references:	
Results (including absolute risk, NNT, etc if possible):	

Question 2:

Cochrane Library search terms used:	Hits

Key references:

Results (including absolute risk, NNT, etc if possible):

PubMed search terms used:	Hits

Key references:

Results (including absolute risk, NNT, etc if possible):

Search results:

Cochrane Library of systematic reviews   no hits

PubMed Clinical Queries (therapy, specific)   1 hit

Scurr et al (2001). Frequency and prevention of symptomless deep-vein thrombosis in long-haul flights: a randomised trial. The Lancet 357:1485–1489.

Authors' conclusion:
'Wearing of elastic compression stockings during long-haul air travel is associated with a reduction in symptomless DVT.'

For this search, we obtained one study, a randomised controlled trial, and the authors concluded that wearing elastic stockings helps to prevent symptomless DVT on long haul flights. But how do we know that the results are valid and real? The full article is included on pages 74–78 of this workbook.

The process that has been developed by biostatisticians and clinical epidemiologists for assessing trials is called '**critical appraisal**'. To critically appraise the article by Scurr et al, we need to consider some important factors that may cause a difference to be observed, either positive or negative, between a treated and control group in a clinical trial. These factors can be summarised as follows:

• whether the groups were representative and comparable

• whether the outcome measurements were accurate

• whether there was a placebo effect

• whether the results were real or could have been due to chance.

The first three points tell us about the **internal validity** of the methods used to conduct the trial. The last point is related to the size and variation in the effect seen in different subjects.

Critical appraisal

Were the groups of subjects representative and comparable?

Setting up representative and comparable groups

If the subjects in a study are not representative of the population to be studied then the outcomes may not be applicable for that population. The best way to ensure that the study groups are representative is to initially select subjects randomly from the whole population of interest, apply relevant inclusion/exclusion criteria and ensure that the study groups are large enough to provide a representative sample (and hence statistically meaningful results).

For comparative studies, once subjects have been recruited for a trial, they must be allocated to either the control or treatment group. If these groups are not as closely matched as possible, then a different outcome for each group may be due to one of the nonmatched characteristics (sometimes called 'confounders') rather than due to the intervention under consideration. Examples of ways in which groups could differ include:

- age
- sex
- socioeconomic group
- smoker/nonsmoker
- disease status
- past exposure to risk factors
- ...... (there are many more)

The best way to ensure that groups are matched is to allocate subjects to them randomly.

However, so-called 'randomisation' can be done very well or rather badly. To be effective, neither the trial subjects, nor the investigators must be able to influence the group each person ends up in (this is called 'allocation concealment'). This is best achieved by using a centralised computer allocation process. This method is usually used for large multicentre trials. For smaller trials, use of an independent person to oversee the allocation (eg the hospital pharmacist) gives a satisfactory result.

Methods such as allocating alternate subjects to each group or handing out sealed envelopes are not as good because the allocation is not as well concealed.

<aside>

Steps in critical appraisal

- were the groups of subjects representative and comparable?

- was the outcome measurement accurate?

- was a placebo used?

- could the results have been due to chance?

</aside>

Other allocation methods are sometimes used, including allocating subjects who present on alternate days or selecting subjects from databases, but these methods do not conceal allocation and are not truly randomised.

Whatever method is used for selection of subjects and group allocation, something unexpected can happen so it is important to check that the groups formed are really closely matched for as many characteristics as possible.

The full article is included on pages 74–78 of this workbook.

How did the DVT trial select and allocate subjects?

Selection

'Volunteers were recruited by placing advertisements in local newspapers....'

'Passengers were included if they were over 50 years of age and intended to travel economy class with two sectors of at least 8 h duration within 6 weeks.'

Volunteers were excluded from the study if they had.......' (various exclusions)

See 'Volunteers and methods: Participants ' (DVT trial p1485)

Allocation

'Volunteers were randomised by sealed envelope to one of two groups'

See 'Volunteers and methods: Randomisation' (DVT trial p1486)

Table 1 Characteristics of study groups (DVT trial p1486)

	No stockings	Stockings
Number	116	115
Pre-study:		
Age	62 (56–68)	61 (56–66)
Females	61 (53%)	81 (70%)*
Varicose veins	41	45
Haemoglobin	142	140
During study:		
Hours flying	22	24
Days of stay	17	16

* $P < 0.01$

Maintaining representative and comparable groups (1): equal treatment

Once comparable groups have been set up at the start of a trial, it is important that they stay that way! The only difference between the two groups should be the treatment being tested. To achieve this, the placebo or control treatment must be given in an identical regimen to the actual treatment.

Did the DVT trial treat subjects equally?

Blood was taken from all participants before travel.

All participants had ultrasonography (US) once before travel (30 had US twice).

Blood was collected from all participants before travel.

All participants were seen within 48 hours of return flight, were interviewed and completed a questionnaire, had a repeat US and a blood sample was taken.

See 'Volunteers and methods; Investigators/Evaluation' (DVT trial pp1485–1486)

Maintaining representative and comparable groups (2): analysis of all subjects

Trial groups may have been carefully randomised to be comparable and they may have received identical treatment in all but the intervention under investigation, but all this is to no avail if some of the subjects leave the trial and are not accounted for in the analysis. This is because the subjects that leave the trial may have a particular characteristic so that those remaining in the groups are no longer matched. This is called the 'intention to treat principle'.

Unequal treatment invalidates results

In a trial of vitamin E in pre-term infants (1948), the vitamin treatment appeared to 'prevent' retrolental fibroplasia. However, this was not due to the vitamin itself but because the babies were on 100% oxygen and the treatment group babies were removed from the oxygen for frequent doses of vitamin, whereas the control babies remained in the oxygen.

'Intention to treat principle'

Once a subject is randomised, he or she should be analysed in the group they are randomised to, even if they never receive treatment, discontinue the trial, or cross over to the other group.

Did the DVT trial follow up all the subjects?

Follow up of subjects

231 subjects were randomised (115 to stockings; 116 none)

200 were analysed

    27 unable to attend for subsequent US

    2 were excluded from analysis because they were upgraded to business class

    2 were excluded from analysis because they were taking anticoagulants

See 'Trial profile' (DVT trial p1486); and 'Results' (pp1486–1487)

How important were the losses?

Were they equally distributed?

    stockings: 15 lost (6 men; 9 women)

    no stockings: 16 lost (7 men, 9 women)

Did they have similar characteristics?

    no other information is provided

Intention-to-treat analysis

'Haematological data were included in the analysis only when volunteers were examined before and after travel. All other analyses were done on an intention-to-treat basis, which included all randomised participants.'

See 'Volunteers and methods: Statistics' (DVT trial p1486)

Was the outcome measurement accurate?

Even if the study groups have been randomly selected and allocated, the results obtained may not reflect the true effect if the outcomes have not been measured accurately. The two most important factors that can affect outcome measurements are:

- measurement bias

- measurement error

Measurement bias

Measurement bias reflects the human tendency to inadvertantly 'nudge' results in the direction that they are predicted to go.

If the subjects know which group they are in then this may affect the way they behave in the trial, comply with the treatment regimen, report their symptoms and so on.

If the person who is making the measurement (outcome assessor) knows which group the subject is in, this can influence the way in which they record the results.

These biases can be overcome by using subjects and outcome assessors that are both 'blinded' to which groups the subjects are allocated to. A trial that is set up this way is called a 'double blind' trial and the results of such a study are least likely to be biased.

A trial in which either the subjects or the outcome assessors are blinded to the group allocation, but not both, is called a single blind study and the results are less reliable than for a double blind study because of the increased potential for bias. A study in which neither the subjects nor the outcome assessors are blinded is the least reliable type of study of all because of the high potential for bias.

Steps in critical appraisal

- were the groups of subjects representative and comparable?

- was the outcome measurement accurate?

- was a placebo used?

- could the results have been due to chance?

'Blinding'

BEST
Double blind trial: subjects and investigators (outcome assessors) both unaware of the group allocations

MODERATE
Single blind trial: either the subject or the investigators are unaware of group allocation

WORST
Not blinded: subjects and investigators both aware of group allocations

> ### How did the DVT trial eliminate measurement bias?
>
>
>
> *Subjects*
>
> 'Although the stockings were allocated randomly, the passengers were aware of the treatment' (ie not blinded)
>
> *See 'Volunteers and methods: Randomisation' (DVT trial p1486)*
>
> *Outcome assessors*
>
> 'Most passengers removed their stockings on completion of their journey. The nurse removed the stockings from those passengers who had continued to wear them. A further duplex examination was then undertaken with the technician unaware of the group to which the volunteer had been randomised' (ie blinded)
>
> *See 'Volunteers and methods: Evaluation' (DVT trial p1486)*

Measurement error

A second problem that can arise for outcome measurements is measurement error. This occurs if outcomes are not measured in the same way for all subjects. It is therefore important to use exactly the same measurement strategy and methods for everyone (both the treatment and control groups).

> ### Was a standardised measurement strategy used for the DVT trial?
>
>
>
> Measurements were carried out using the same procedures for all volunteers.
>
> *See 'Volunteers and methods: Investigators' (DVT trial p1485); and 'Evaluation' (p1486)*

Measurement error

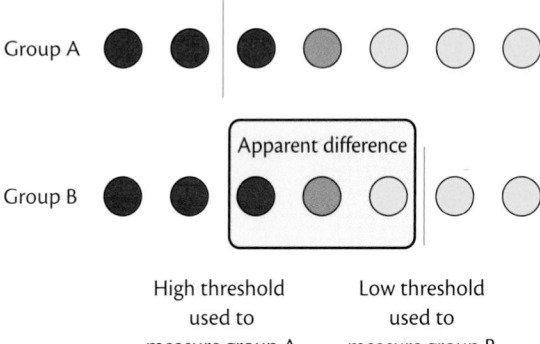

Was a placebo used?

The 'placebo effect' is the so-called effect that is attributable to the expectation that the treatment will have an effect.

Placebo effect — Trial in patients with chronic severe itching

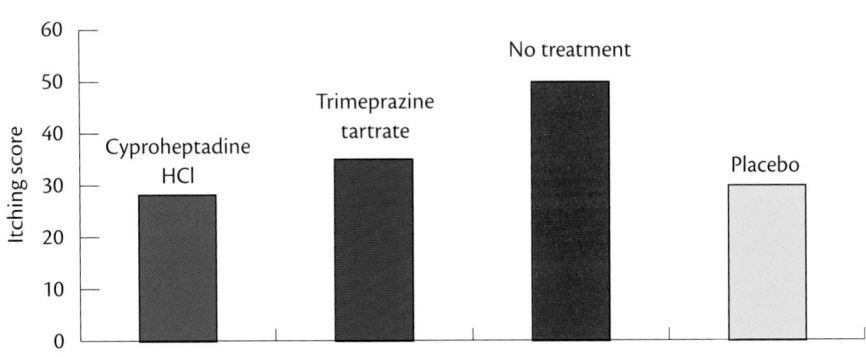

Treatment vs no treatment vs placebo for itching

Steps in critical appraisal

- were the groups of subjects representative and comparable?
- was the outcome measurement accurate?
- was a placebo used?
- could the results have been due to chance?

Thus, in a trial where a treatment is compared with no treatment, an effect (even quite a large one) may be due to the 'placebo effect', rather that to the effect of the treatment itself. This means that whenever it is practical to do so, the control group in an RCT should receive a placebo treatment (eg a sugar pill, or sham procedure) that is indistinguishable from the real thing.

Did the DVT trial use a placebo?

In the DVT trial, volunteers were randomised to two groups, one with and one without elastic stockings. The volunteers who did not receive elastic stockings were not provided with a substitute treatment (placebo).

See 'Volunteers and methods: Randomisation' (DVT trial p1486)

Could the results have been due to chance?

We can never determine the true risk of an outcome in a population. The best we can do is estimate the true risk based on the sample of subjects in a trial. This is called the point estimate. How do we know that the point estimate from the trial reflects the true population risk?

This is where statistics comes in. We will not go into the statistical methods used here but, suffice it to say, that statistics provides two methods of assessing chance:

* *P*-values (hypothesis testing)
* confidence intervals (estimation)

P-values are a measure of probability. Most research is about testing a 'null hypothesis' (which means a hypothesis that there will not be an effect). If there is an effect (ie the null hypothesis is disproved), the *P*-value tells us the probability that this was due to chance alone. For example, if the *P*-value is less than 0.05, it means that the probability that the result was due to chance is less than 5%. This means that we would have to repeat the study 20 times (100/5) for there to be an even chance of the effect occurring by chance alone. This is called a statistically significant result.

Confidence intervals (CIs) are an estimate of the range of values that are likely to include the real value. If the CIs for the treatment and control groups are small and do not overlap, we can be pretty sure that the result is real. If the CIs are large and overlapping, we cannot be nearly as confident about what the real result is.

Steps in critical appraisal

* were the groups of subjects representative and comparable?
* was the outcome measurement accurate?
* was a placebo used?
* could the results have been due to chance?

What were the results of the DVT trial?

DVT in stocking group
0 (0%; 95% CI 0–3.2%)

DVT in control group
12 (10%; 95% CI 4.8–16%)

P-value   Not quoted in the paper; but results are statistically significant because CI values do not overlap.

See 'Results' (DVT trial p 1487)

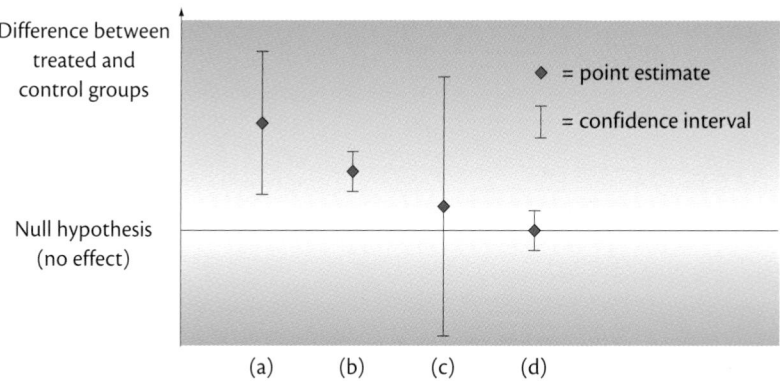

(a)   Statistically significant result (P < 0.05) but low precision
(b)   Statistically significant result (P < 0.05) with high precision
(c)   Not statistically significant result (P > 0.05) with low precision
(d)   Not statistically significant result (no effect) with high precision

However, an intervention can only be considered useful if the 95% CI includes clinically important treatment effects. An important distinction therefore needs to be made between statistical significance and clinical importance:

- statistical significance relates to the size of the effect and the 95% CIs in relation to the null hypothesis

- clinical importance relates to the size of the effect and the 95% CIs in relation to a minimum effect that would be considered to be clinically important.

For example, a reduction in a symptom may be measurable and statistically significant, but unless it is sufficient to avoid the need for medication or improve the quality of life of the patient, then it may not be considered clinically important.

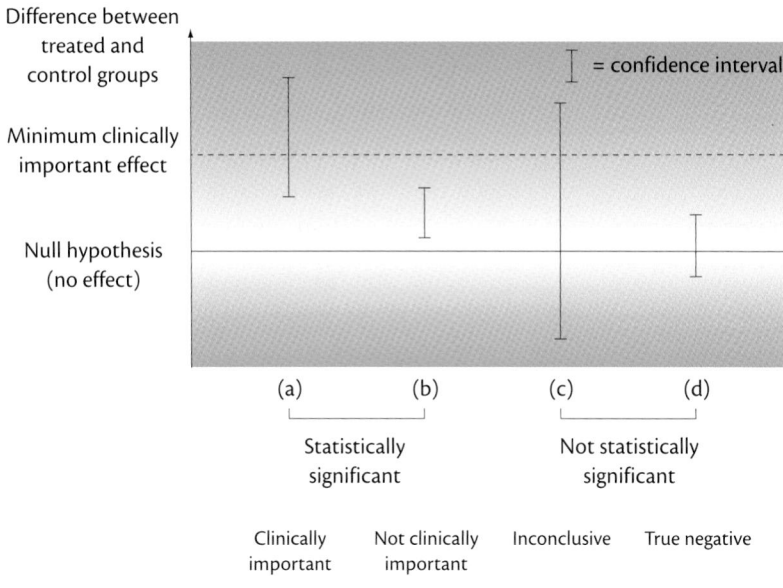

(a)   Difference is statistically significant and clinically important
(b)   Difference is statistically significant but not clinically important
(c)   Difference is not statistically significant and of uncertain clinical importance
(d)   Difference is not statistically significant and not clinically important

Outcome measures

Most often the results are presented as dichotomous outcomes (ie 'yes' or 'no' outcomes that either happen or don't happen) such as cancer, heart attack or death.

Consider a study in which 15% (0.15) of the control group and 10% (0.10) of the treatment group died after 2 years of treatment. The results can be expressed in many ways as shown below*.

Measure	Meaning	Example*
Relative risk(RR) = risk of outcome in the treatment group divided by the risk of outcome in the control group	RR tells us how many times more likely it is that an event will occur in the treatment group relative to the control group. RR = 1 means that there is no difference between the 2 groups RR < 1 means that the treatment reduced the risk of the outcome RR > 1 means that the treatment increased the risk of the outcome	RR = 0.1/0.15 = 0.67 Since RR< 1, the treatment decreases the risk of death.
Absolute risk reduction (ARR) = risk of outcome in the control group minus risk of outcome in the treatment group (also known as the absolute risk difference)	ARR tells us the absolute difference in the rates of events between the two groups and gives an indication of the baseline risk and treatment effect. ARR = 0 means that there is no difference between the 2 groups (thus, the treatment had no effect)	ARR = 0.15-0.10 = 0.05 (5%) The absolute benefit of treatment is a 5% reduction in the death rate.
Relative risk reduction (RRR) = ARR divided by the risk of outcome in control group (or, 1 – RR)	RRR tells us the reduction in rate of the outcome in the treatment group relative to the control group. RRR is probably the most commonly reported measure of treatment effects.	RRR = 0.05/0.15 = 0.33 (33%) OR 1–0.67 = 0.33 (33%)
Number needed to treat (NNT) = 1/ARR	NNT tells us the number of patients we need to treat with the treatment under consideration in order to prevent 1 bad outcome.	NNT = 1/0.05 = 20 We would need to treat 20 people for 2 years in order to prevent 1 death.

Summary of critical appraisal of DVT trial

Internal validity

In the DVT trial, subjects were initially selected on a volunteer basis. Inclusion/ exclusion criteria ensured that the recruited subjects were representative of the population of interest (over 50, travelling long distance by economy class, no previous history of DVT, etc). Although not a very large study, the number of subjects (approximately 100 per group) was sufficient to provide a representative sample (and hence statistically meaningful results).

Group allocation was random but the method used (sealed envelope) was not a very effective method for eliminating allocation bias.

Either due to allocation bias (were women more prepared to wear elastic stockings?) or other factors, there was a statistically significant difference in sex ratio between the groups. The groups were well matched for other factors.

Once allocated to groups, all subjects were treated equally in the trial and there were only a few losses to follow up.

The trial was single blinded (subjects were aware of whether they were wearing stockings or not, but outcome assessors were not). Outcomes were measured using the same methodology for both groups. The control group did not receive a placebo treatment.

Conclusion: The trial was moderately well conducted but had some methodological flaws that could have affected the outcomes.

Results

The results showed a large difference between the treated and control groups with no overlap in CIs.

Absolute risk reduction (ARR)   = 0.10 (10%)

NNT   = 1/0.10 = 10

Overall conclusion

While the results show a reduction in symptomless DVT in long-haul air passengers, the study had some design flaws that would warrant further investigation of this issue.

Frequency and prevention of symptomless deep-vein thrombosis in long-haul flights: a randomised trial

John H Scurr, Samuel J Machin, Sarah Bailey-King, Ian J Mackie, Sally McDonald, Philip D Coleridge Smith

Summary

Background The true frequency of deep-vein thrombosis (DVT) during long-haul air travel is unknown. We sought to determine the frequency of DVT in the lower limb during long-haul economy-class air travel and the efficacy of graduated elastic compression stockings in its prevention.

Methods We recruited 89 male and 142 female passengers over 50 years of age with no history of thromboembolic problems. Passengers were randomly allocated to one of two groups: one group wore class-I below-knee graduated elastic compression stockings, the other group did not. All the passengers made journeys lasting more than 8 h per flight (median total duration 24 h), returning to the UK within 6 weeks. Duplex ultrasonography was used to assess the deep veins before and after travel. Blood samples were analysed for two specific common gene mutations, factor V Leiden (FVL) and prothrombin G20210A (PGM), which predispose to venous thromboembolism. A sensitive D-dimer assay was used to screen for the development of recent thrombosis.

Findings 12/116 passengers (10%; 95% CI 4·8–16·0%) developed symptomless DVT in the calf (five men, seven women). None of these passengers wore elastic compression stockings, and two were heterozygous for FVL. Four further patients who wore elastic compression stockings, had varicose veins and developed superficial thrombophlebitis. One of these passengers was heterozygous for both FVL and PGM. None of the passengers who wore class-I compression stockings developed DVT (95% CI 0–3·2%).

Interpretation We conclude that symptomless DVT might occur in up to 10% of long-haul airline travellers. Wearing of elastic compression stockings during long-haul air travel is associated with a reduction in symptomless DVT.

Lancet 2001; **357:** 1485–89

See Commentary page 1461

Department of Surgery (J H Scurr FRCS, P D Coleridge Smith FRCS) **and Department of Haematology** (Prof S J Machin FRCP, I J Mackie PhD, S McDonald BSc), **Royal Free and University College Medical School, London, UK; and Stamford Hospital, London, UK** (S Bailey-King RCN)

Correspondence to: Mr J H Scurr, Lister Hospital, Chelsea Bridge Road, London SW1W 8RH, UK
(e-mail: medleg@mailbox.co.uk)

Introduction

Every year the number of passengers travelling over long distances by air increases. Physicians working close to major airports have seen individual cases presenting with thromboembolic problems after air travel.[1-3] Results of retrospective clinical series[4-6] suggest that up to 20% of patients presenting with thromboembolism have undertaken recent air travel. Ferrari et al[7] reported a strong association between deep-vein thrombosis (DVT) and long travel (>4 h) in a case-control study, although only a quarter of his patients with DVT travelled by air. Kraaijenhagen and colleagues[8] looked at travel in the previous 4 weeks in patients presenting with DVT. They concluded that travelling times of more than 5 h were not associated with increased risk of DVT. The true frequency of this problem remains unknown and controversial. Episodes of DVT can arise without any symptom. Less than half the patients with symptomless DVT will develop symptoms, and only a few of those go on to have a clinically detectable pulmonary embolism.[9,10] In surgical series, a link between symptomless DVT, symptomatic DVT, and pulmonary embolism has been established.[11,12] Patients undergoing surgical procedures are assessed for risk, and appropriate prophylaxis is implemented.[13] We undertook a randomised controlled trial to assess the overall frequency of DVT in long-haul airline passengers and the efficacy of a class-I elastic compression stocking for the duration of the flight.

Volunteers and methods

Participants

Volunteers were recruited by placing advertisements in local newspapers and travel shops, and by press releases. The Aviation Health Institute referred many of the volunteers initially screened for this study, which took place in the Vascular Institute at the Stamford Hospital, London, UK. Passengers were included if they were over 50 years of age and intended to travel economy class with two sectors of at least 8 h duration within 6 weeks. Passengers were invited to undergo preliminary screening, which included an examination and completion of a medical questionnaire about previous illnesses and medication. Volunteers were excluded from the study if they had had episodes of venous thrombosis, were taking anticoagulants, regularly wore compression stockings, had cardiorespiratory problems, or had any other serious illness, including malignant disease. The study was approved by Stamford Hospital ethics committee. Volunteers who gave informal written consent were included in the study.

Investigators

Volunteers who were eligible for inclusion were investigated by duplex ultrasonography (General Electric LOGIQ 700, GE Medical Systems, Waukesha, USA) to detect evidence of previous venous thrombosis. The lower limbs were assessed by two technicians skilled in assessment of venous problems. Examinations were done with volunteers standing. To assess the competence of deep and superficial veins the technicians manually compressed the calf and measured the duration of reverse flow by colour or pulsed doppler sonography. Venous reflux was defined as duration of reverse flow exceeding 0·5 s. The presence of current or previous venous thrombosis was assessed from the B-mode image, colour flow mapping, and compression assessment of veins during B-mode imaging. Passengers who had evidence of previous thrombosis were excluded.

In the first 30 volunteers, ultrasound examination was undertaken 2 weeks before air travel and again within 2 days of the start of the first flight to provide a control interval in which occurrence of spontaneous DVT could be assessed in this population. No acute DVT was detected during this period. The logistics of the study made it difficult for passengers to attend Stamford Hospital on two occasions before travel and this part of the investigation was abandoned in the remaining volunteers. All subsequent volunteers were screened once before they travelled.

Blood was taken from all participants before travel for a series of haemostatic tests. Full blood and platelet counts were done on a routine cell counter. We used the Dimertest Gold EIA assay (Agen Biomedical Ltd, Acacia Ridge, Australia) to measure D-dimer. We took the upper 95% confidence limit of normal value as 120 pg/L. We used routine PCR techniques for identification of the factor V Leiden and prothrombin G20210A gene mutations.

Randomisation

Volunteers were randomised by sealed envelope to one of two groups. The control group received no specific additional treatment; the other group was given class-I (German Hohenstein compression standard; 20–30 mm Hg) below-knee elastic compression stockings (Mediven Travel; Medi UK Ltd, Hereford, UK). Participants were advised to put on the stockings before the start of travel and to remove the stockings after arrival for every flight by which they travelled. Although the stockings were allocated randomly, the passengers were aware of the treatment. Passengers arranged their own air travel. There was no collaboration with the airlines, although two passengers were upgraded from economy to business class.

Evaluation

Passengers reattended the Stamford Hospital within 48 h of their return flight. They were interviewed by a research nurse and completed a questionnaire inquiring about: duration of air travel, wearing of stockings, symptoms in the lower limbs, and illnesses and medication taken during their trip. Most passengers removed their stockings on completion of their journey. The nurse removed the stockings from those passengers who had continued to wear them. A further duplex examination was then undertaken with the technician unaware of the group to which the volunteer had been randomised. Another blood sample was taken for repeat D-dimer assay. In passengers for whom clinically significant abnormalities of the lower limb veins were detected on duplex ultrasonography, including calf vein thrombosis, the volunteers' general practitioners were notified in writing so that treatment could be arranged.

Statistics

Because of insufficient published data we could not pre-calculate sample size. Since the investigation was intended as a pilot study, we chose a total of 200 passengers. Recruitment was continued until 100 volunteers had been investigated in each group. A finding

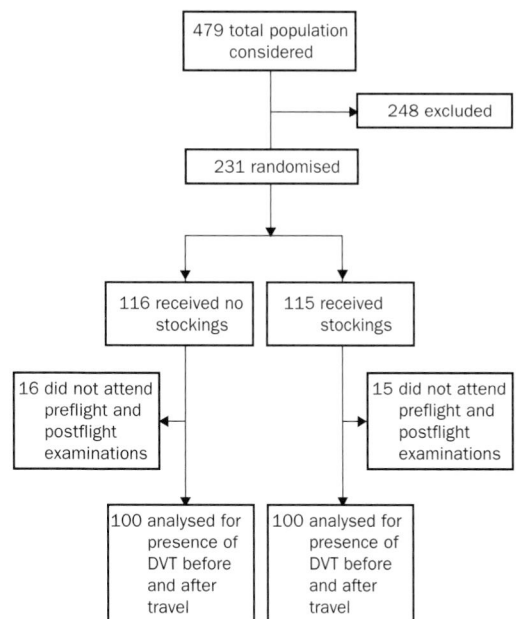

Trial profile

of no case of venous thrombosis in this number of passengers would have resulted in a 95% CI for the rate of DVT of 0–2%. To measure a thrombotic event occurring in 2% or fewer passengers would require a very large study, and the low frequency would have limited implications for air travellers. Data were analysed by contingency tables and calculation of the differences in proportions, and 95% CIs by a computer program (CIA version 1.1, 1989, BMA Publishers, London, UK). We used median and interquartile range for haematological data since data were not normally distributed. Haematological data were included in the analysis only when volunteers were examined before and after travel. All other analyses were done on an intention-to-treat basis, which included all randomised participants.

Results

Volunteers were excluded before randomisation if they did not fulfil the entry requirements or could not attend hospital for investigation both before and after travel (figure). Thus, 231 of 479 volunteers were randomised. 27 passengers were unable to attend for subsequent ultrasound investigation because of ill-health (three), change of travel plans, or inability to keep appointments (24). Two who

	No stockings	Stockings
Number	116	115
Age (years)	62 (56–68)	61 (56–66)
Number of women (%)	61 (53%)	81 (70%)
Number with varicose veins	41	45
Days of stay	17 (13–32)	16 (13–27)
Hours flying time	22 (18–36)	24 (19–35)
Haemoglobin (g/L)	142 (133–149)	140 (133–147)
WBC (×10⁹/L)	5·9 (5·0–7·3)	6·0 (5·0–6·9)
Packed cell volume	0·44 (0·42–0·47)	0·44 (0·41–0·46)
Platelets (×10⁹/L)	240 (206–272)	242 (219–290)
Number FVL positive	7	4
Number PGM positive	1	3

Median (interquartile range) shown, unless otherwise indicated. WBC=white blood cells. FVL=factor V Leiden. PGM=prothrombin gene mutation.

Table 1: **Characteristics of study groups**

Reproduced for this workbook with permission from Elsevier.

8   Kraaijenhagen RA, Haverkamp D, Koopman MMW, Prandoni P, Piovella F, Büller H. Travel and the risk of venous thrombosis. *Lancet* 2000; **356:** 1492–93.

9   Kakkar VV, Howe CT, Flanc C, Clarke MB. Natural history of postoperative deep-vein thrombosis. *Lancet* 1969; **2:** 230–32.

10 Negus D, Pinto DJ. Natural history of postoperative deep-vein thrombosis. *Lancet* 1969; **2:** 645.

11 Dalen JE, Alpert JS. Natural history of pulmonary embolism. *Prog Cardiovasc Dis* 1975; **17:** 259–70.

12 Coon WW. Epidemiology of venous thromboembolism. *Ann Surg* 1977; **186:** 149–64.

13 THRIFT Consensus Group. Risk of and prophylaxis for venous thromboembolism in hospital patients. Thromboembolic Risk Factors. *BMJ* 1992; **305:** 567–74.

14 Collins R, Scrimgeour A, Yusuf S, Peto R. Reduction in fatal pulmonary embolism and venous thrombosis by perioperative administration of subcutaneous heparin. Overview of results of randomized trials in general, orthopaedic, and urologic surgery. *N Engl J Med* 1988; **318:** 1162–73.

15 Kazmers A, Groehn H, Meeker C. Acute calf vein thrombosis: outcomes and implications. *Am Surg* 1999; **65:** 1124–27.

16 O'Shaughnessy AM, Fitzgerald DE. The value of duplex ultrasound in the follow-up of acute calf vein thrombosis. *Int Angiol* 1997; **16:** 142–46.

17 Meissner MH, Caps MT, Bergelin RO, Manzo RA, Strandness DE Jr. Early outcome after isolated calf vein thrombosis. *J Vasc Surg* 1997; **26:** 749–56.

18 Colditz GA, Tuden RL, Oster G. Rates of venous thrombosis after general surgery: combined results of randomised clinical trials. *Lancet* 1986; **2:** 143–46.

19 Bounameaux H, de Moerloose P, Perrier A, Reber G. Plasma measurement of D-dimer as a diagnostic aid in suspected venous thromboembolism: an overview. *Thromb Haemost* 1994; **71:** 1–6.

20 Bendz B, Rostrup M, Sevre K, Andersen T, Sandset PM. Association between acute hypobaric hypoxia and activation of coagulation in human beings. *Lancet* 2000; **356:** 1657–58.

21 Nicolaides AN, Irving D. Clinical factors and the risk of deep vein thrombosis. In: Nicolaides AN, ed. Thromboembolism: aetiology, advances in prevention and management. Lancaster: MTP, 1975: 193–203.

22 Kniffin WD Jr, Baron JA, Barrett J, Birkmeyer JD, Anderson FA Jr. The epidemiology of diagnosed pulmonary embolism and deep venous thrombosis in the elderly. *Arch Intern Med* 1994; **154:** 861–66.

23 Robinson KS, Anderson DR, Gross M, et al. Accuracy of screening compression ultrasonography and clinical examination for the diagnosis of deep vein thrombosis after total hip or knee arthroplasty. *Can J Surg* 1998; **41:** 368–73.

24 Cornuz J, Pearson SD, Polak JF. Deep venous thrombosis: complete lower extremity venous US evaluation in patients without known risk factors—outcome study. *Radiology* 1999; **211:** 637–41.

25 Westrich GH, Allen ML, Tarantino SJ, et al. Ultrasound screening for deep venous thrombosis after total knee athroplasty. 2-year reassessment. *Clin Orthop* 1998; **356:** 125–33.

26 Forbes K, Stevenson AJ. The use of power Doppler ultrasound in the diagnosis of isolated deep venous thrombosis of the calf. *Clin Radiol* 1998; **53:** 752–54.

27 Mantoni M, Strandberg C, Neergaard K, et al. Triplex US in the diagnosis of asymptomatic deep venous thrombosis. *Acta Radiol* 1997; **38:** 327–31.

28 Robertson PL, Goergen SK, Waugh JR, Fabiny RP. Colour-assisted compression ultrasound in the diagnosis of calf deep venous thrombosis. *Med J Aust* 1995; **163:** 515–18.

29 Krunes U, Teubner K, Knipp H, Holzapfel R. Thrombosis of the muscular calf veins-reference to a syndrome which receives little attention. *Vasa* 1998; **27:** 172–75.

Critical appraisal of your own trial

Now you can critically appraise one of the articles about an intervention that you identified during your earlier search session or the article on immunisation of infants that is included at the end of this section (see pages 83–85).

For the chosen article, work through the critical appraisal sheet on the next pages and then:

(a) decide whether the internal validity of the study is sufficient to allow firm conclusions (all studies have some flaws; but are these flaws bad enough to discard the study?)

(b) if the study is sufficiently valid, look at and interpret the results — what is the relevance or size of the effects of the intervention?

B. RESULTS

1. What measure was used and how large was the treatment effect?

2. Could the effect have been due to chance?	
P-value	
Confidence interval (CI)	

CONCLUSION

Internal validity:

Results:

Funding: This work was undertaken while MJ was visiting scholar to the department of family practice, University of British Columbia, Canada. He was funded by the department of primary care and population sciences, Royal Free and University College Medical Schools, University College London, NHS prolonged study leave, and a grant from the King's Fund.

Competing interests: None declared.

1 Department of Health. *NHS primary care walk in centres*. London: DoH, 1999 (HSC 1999/116).
2 Wilkie P, Logan A. Walk in centres. *Br J Gen Pract* 2000;49:1017.
3 Shah CP. *Public health and preventive medicine in Canada*. Toronto: University of Toronto Press, 1994.
4 Feldman W, Cullum C. The pediatric walk-in clinic. *CMAJ* 1984;130:1003-5.
5 Miller GB, Mah Z, Nantes S, Bryant W, Kayler T, McKinnon K. Ontario walk in clinics. *Can Fam Physician* 1989;35:2013-5.
6 Rizos J, Anglin P, Grava-Gubins I, Lazar C. Walk-in clinics. *CMAJ* 1990;143:740-5.
7 Bell NR, Szafran O. Use of walk in clinics by family practice patients. *Can Fam Physician* 1992;38:507-13.
8 Rachlis V. Who goes to after-hours clinics? *Can Fam Physician* 1993;39:226-70.
9 Burnett MG, Grover SA. Use of the emergency department for non-urgent care. *CMAJ* 1996;154:1345-51.
10 Grad R, Kaczorowski J, Singer Y, Levitt C, Mandelcorn J. Where do family practice patients go in case of emergency? *Can Fam Physician* 1998;44:2666-72.
11 Weinkauf DJ, Kralj B. Medical service provision and costs. *Can Public Policy* 1998;24:471-84.
12 Szafran O, Bell NR. Use of walk in clinics by rural and urban patients. *Can Fam Physician* 2000;46:114-9.
13 Miller GB, Nantes S. Walk in clinics and primary care. *Can Fam Physician* 1989;35:2019-22.
14 Borkenhagen RH. Walk in clinics. *Can Fam Physician* 1996;42:1879-83.
15 Milne P. Could you compete with a walk-in clinic? *CMAJ* 1987;136:534.
16 What's wrong with walk-ins? *CMAJ* 1988;139:63-4.
17 Burak AJ. Walk in clinics. *Br Columbia Coll Fam Physicians* 1994; October:5-6.
18 Makin MD. McDonald's medicine. *Br Columbia Med J* 1993;35:151.
19 Milne M. Walk-in clinics. *CMAJ* 1987;137:532-6.
20 Rizos J. Walk-in clinics. *CMAJ* 1991;144:631-2.
21 Rowlands J. After hours clinics. *Ont Med Rev* 1988;55:10-7.
22 Wishart D. BC GPs unite to fight walk in clinics. *CMAJ* 1987;137:535.
23 Toews B. Walk in clinics add to costs. *Br Columbia Med J* 1992;34:202.

(Accepted 10 July 2000)

Effect of needle length on incidence of local reactions to routine immunisation in infants aged 4 months: randomised controlled trial

Linda Diggle, Jonathan Deeks

Abstract

Objective To compare rates of local reactions associated with two needle sizes used to administer routine immunisations to infants.

Design Randomised controlled trial.

Setting Routine immunisation clinics in eight general practices in Buckinghamshire.

Participants Healthy infants attending for third primary immunisation due at 16 weeks of age: 119 infants were recruited, and 110 diary cards were analysed.

Interventions Immunisation with 25 gauge, 16 mm, orange hub needle or 23 gauge, 25 mm, blue hub needle.

Main outcome measures Parental recordings of redness, swelling, and tenderness for three days after immunisation.

Results Rate of redness with the longer needle was initially two thirds the rate with the smaller needle (relative risk 0.66 (95% confidence interval 0.45 to 0.99), $P = 0.04$), and by the third day this had decreased to a seventh (relative risk 0.13 (0.03 to 0.56), $P = 0.0006$). Rate of swelling with the longer needle was initially about a third that with the smaller needle (relative risk 0.39 (0.23 to 0.67), $P = 0.0002$), and this difference remained for all three days. Rates of tenderness were also lower with the longer needle throughout follow up, but not significantly (relative risk 0.60 (0.29 to 1.25), $P = 0.17$).

Conclusions Use of 25 mm needles significantly reduced rates of local reaction to routine infant immunisation. On average, for every five infants vaccinated, use of the longer needle instead of the shorter needle would prevent one infant from experiencing any local reaction. Vaccine manufacturers should review their policy of supplying the shorter needle in vaccine packs.

Introduction

As part of the UK childhood immunisation schedule, infants routinely receive diphtheria, pertussis, and tetanus (DPT) vaccine and *Haemophilus influenzae* type b (Hib) vaccine at 2, 3, and 4 months.[1] Nationally available guidelines advise practitioners to administer primary vaccines to infants by deep subcutaneous or intramuscular injection using either a 25 or 23 gauge needle but give no recommendation regarding needle length.[1] The question of optimum needle length for infant immunisation has not previously been addressed in Britain, despite calls from nurses for evidence on which to base immunisation practice. We conducted a randomised controlled trial of the two needle sizes currently used by UK practitioners to determine whether needle size affects the incidence of redness, swelling, and tenderness.

Participants and methods

Participants

Eight of 11 general practices approached in Buckinghamshire agreed to participate in the study. Practice nurses recruited healthy infants attending routine immunisation clinics. Parents received written information about the study when attending for the second primary vaccination and were asked if they wished to participate when they returned for the third vaccination. The only exclusion criteria were those normally applicable to a child receiving primary immunisations.[1]

Oxford Vaccine Group, University Department of Paediatrics, John Radcliffe Hospital, Oxford OX3 9DU
Linda Diggle
senior research nurse

ICRF/NHS Centre for Statistics in Medicine, Institute of Health Sciences, University of Oxford, Oxford OX3 7LF
Jonathan Deeks
senior medical statistician

Correspondence to:
L Diggle
linda.diggle@paediatrics.oxford.ac.uk

BMJ 2000;321:931–3

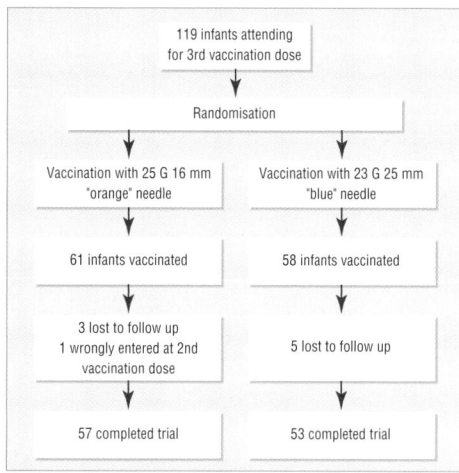

Flow chart describing randomisation sequence

We obtained ethical approval from the local ethics committee.

Interventions

Infants were allocated to receive their third primary immunisation with either the 25 gauge, 16 mm needle or the 23 gauge, 25 mm needle according to a computer generated blocked randomisation scheme stratified

by practice. Allocations were concealed in sequentially numbered opaque envelopes opened once written parental consent was obtained. Practice nurses were instructed verbally, by demonstration and in writing, to use the technique of injecting into the anterolateral thigh, stretching the skin taut and inserting the needle at a 90° angle to the skin.[2] The right thigh was used, with the needle inserted into the skin up to the hub.

Outcomes

Parents recorded redness, swelling, and tenderness in a diary for three days after immunisation. The size of swelling and redness were measured with a plastic ruler, while the child's reaction to movement of the limb or to touch of the site was graded with a standard scale. We supplied parents with a prepaid envelope to return the diary, and we contacted parents by telephone if return was delayed.

At the start of the trial all practices were using the 0.5 ml mix of Pasteur-Merieux DPT/Hib vaccine. However, a change in national vaccine supply necessitated a switch to the 1.0 ml mix of Evans DPT and Wyeth Lederle Hib-Titer. Blocked randomisation ensured that the numbers receiving each vaccine were evenly distributed between the groups.

Statistical analysis

In order to detect clinically important relative differences of 25% in tenderness and 30% in redness

Baseline characteristics of 4 month old infants and rate of local reactions to immunisation over three days by needle used for vaccination. Values are numbers (percentages) of infants unless stated otherwise

Local reaction	Size of needle		Difference between longer and shorter needle	
	23 G, 25 mm (n=53)	25 G, 16 mm (n=57)	Relative risk (95% CI); P value	Test for trend
Baseline characteristics				
Mean (SD) weight (kg)*	6.7 (0.9)	6.8 (0.9)		
Age at vaccination (weeks):				
16-17	37 (70)	36 (63)		
18-19	11 (21)	16 (28)		
≥20	5 (9)	5 (9)		
Sex				
Male	34 (64)	30 (53)		
Female	19 (36)	27 (47)		
Site of injection:				
Left leg	13 (25)	12 (21)		
Right leg	40 (75)	45 (79)		
Vaccine type†:				
0.5 ml	8 (15)	8 (14)		
1.0 ml	45 (85)	49 (86)		
Local reactions				
Redness:				
At 6 hours	21 (40)	34 (60)	0.66 (0.45 to 0.99); P=0.04	P=0.007
At 1 day	15 (28)	36 (63)	0.45 (0.28 to 0.72); P=0.0002	P<0.0001
At 2 days	5 (9)	22 (39)	0.24 (0.10 to 0.60); P=0.0004	P=0.0004
At 3 days	2 (4)	16 (28)	0.13 (0.03 to 0.56); P=0.0006	P=0.001
Swelling:				
At 6 hours	12 (23)	33 (58)	0.39 (0.23 to 0.67); P=0.0002	P=0.0009
At 1 day	15 (28)	36 (63)	0.45 (0.28 to 0.72); P=0.0002	P=0.0001
At 2 days	10 (19)	29 (51)	0.37 (0.20 to 0.69); P=0.0005	P=0.0007
At 3 days	7 (13)	23 (40)	0.33 (0.15 to 0.70); P=0.001	P=0.002
Tenderness:				
At 6 hours	9 (17)	16 (28)	0.60 (0.29 to 1.25); P=0.17	P=0.4
At 1 day	4 (8)	8 (14)	0.54 (0.17 to 1.68); P=0.3	P=0.4
At 2 days	0	3 (5)	0 (not estimable); P=0.09	P=0.4
At 3 days	0	1 (2)	0 (not estimable); P=0.3	P=0.2
Any local reaction	33 (62)	48 (84)	0.74 (0.58 to 0.94); P=0.009	

*Weight missing for three infants.
†0.5 ml vaccine=Pasteur Merieux DPT/Hib. 1 ml vaccine=Evans DPT reconstituting Wyeth Lederle Hib-Titer.

and swelling, we estimated that 250 infants should be recruited for the study to have 80% power of detecting differences at the 5% significance level. In January 2000, problems with vaccine supply necessitated the temporary nationwide replacement of the whole cell component of the combined DPT/Hib vaccine with acellular pertussis vaccine.[3] As this vaccine has a different local reactogenicity profile, we decided to stop the trial early.

We used χ^2 tests to compare the proportions of children with each local reaction at 6 hours and 1, 2, and 3 days after immunisation. We compared differences in the size of reaction using a χ^2 test for trend.

Results

Of the 119 children recruited to the study, 61 were randomised to the 16 mm needle group and 58 to the 25 mm needle group (see figure). Nine were not included in the analysis (four in the 16 mm needle group and five in the 25 mm group): diaries were not returned for eight, while the ninth was mistakenly included in the study at the second vaccination. Inclusion of this child did not materially affect the results. The two groups had similar baseline characteristics (see table).

Over half of the infants vaccinated with the 16 mm needle subsequently experienced redness and swelling (table). The rate of redness with the 25 mm needle was initially two thirds the rate with the 16 mm needle (relative risk 0.66 (95% confidence interval 0.45 to 0.99)), and, by the third day, this had decreased further to a seventh (relative risk 0.13 (0.03 to 0.56)). Similarly, rates of swelling after injection with the longer needle were initially around a third of those after use of the smaller needle (relative risk 0.39 (0.23 to 0.67)), and this difference was maintained for all three days. These differences were statistically significant. Tenderness was less frequent and, although the rates of tenderness were also lower with the longer needle throughout follow up, the differences were not significant (table).

Discussion

This study showed that both redness and swelling were significantly reduced when the 23 gauge, 25 mm, blue hub needle was used instead of the 25 gauge, 16 mm, orange hub needle to administer the third dose of diphtheria, pertussis, and tetanus and *Haemophilus influenzae* type b vaccines to infants. The differences suggest that, for every three to five infants vaccinated with the longer rather than the shorter needle, one case of redness and one of swelling would be prevented.

The needles compared in this study are those most commonly used in general practice.[4] As they differed in both length (16 v 25 mm) and bore (25 v 23 gauge), we cannot know which of these factors determined the observed differences in the rates of redness and swelling. However, previous studies comparing injections given at different depths (subcutaneous versus intramuscular) with the same gauge needle have shown similar differences in local reactions.[5 6] We suggest that the length of the longer needle used in our

What is already known on this topic

Most infants experience local reactions to routine vaccinations

Previous local reactions have been cited by parents as a disincentive to further vaccinations

National guidelines on immunisation do not specify a preferred needle length

What this study adds

Local reactions are significantly reduced by use of the 23 gauge, 25 mm, blue hub needle rather than the 25 gauge, 16 mm, orange hub needle supplied by vaccine manufacturers

study ensured that the vaccine reached the thigh muscle in 4 month old infants.

Although our study was not blinded, parents were not told which needle was used to vaccinate their child. We believe that if knowledge of needle allocation introduced bias into the results, it would be less likely that such bias would be in the direction of the longer needle.

These findings are of clinical importance for those involved in administering infant immunisations. In the United Kingdom, where routine vaccines are currently supplied with the shorter needle, a change in the manufacturing process is now required. Any factor that can reduce the rates of adverse reactions in childhood vaccinations has the potential to improve parental acceptance of vaccines[7] and would be welcomed by practitioners.

We thank the parents and babies involved in the study, and the following practice nurses at Buckinghamshire surgeries for recruiting infants and administering immunisations: Lyn Hurry, Waddesdon; Lyn Murphy, Whitehill; Carol Gill, Aston Clinton; Judith Brown, Meadowcroft; Cesca Carter, Wendover; Nicky Oliver, Oakfield; Chris Mildred, Wing; Clare Stroud, Tring Road. We also thank Professor Richard Moxon and Drs Paul Heath, Jim Buttery, Jodie McVernon, Jenny MacLennan, and Karen Sleeman from the Oxford Vaccine Group for helpful advice and support and Dr Ann Mulhall for research supervision.

Contributors: LD conceived and planned the study, recruited and trained practice nurses, managed data collection, wrote the first draft of the paper, and is guarantor for the study. JD advised on design, produced the randomisation scheme, and undertook all analyses. Both authors had input into the final manuscript.

Funding: This study was funded by the Smith and Nephew Foundation through the award of a nursing research scholarship.

Competing interests: None declared.

1 Department of Health. *Immunisation against infectious diseases.* London: HMSO, 1996.
2 World Health Organisation. *Immunisation in practice. Module 8. During a session: giving immunisations.* Geneva: WHO, 1998. (www.who.int/vaccines-documents/DoxTrng/H4IIP.htm (accessed 3 October 2000).)
3 Department of Health. *Current vaccine issues: action update.* London: DoH, 1999. (Professional letter PL/CMO/99/5.)
4 Diggle L. A randomised controlled trial of different needle lengths on the incidence of local reactions when administering the combined injection of diphtheria/pertussis/tetanus (DPT) and Haemophilus influenzae type b (Hib) to infants at 4-months of age [dissertation]. London: Royal College of Nursing Institute, 1999.
5 Mark A, Carlsson R, Granstrom M. Subcutaneous versus intramuscular injection for booster DT vaccination of adolescents. *Vaccine* 1999;17:2067-72.
6 Scheifele DW, Bjornson G, Boraston S. Local adverse effects of meningococcal vaccine. *Can Med Assoc J* 1994;150:14-5.
7 Lieu T, Black S, Ray G, Martin K, Shinefield H, Weniger B. The hidden costs of infant vaccination. *Vaccine* 2000;19:33-41.

(Accepted 22 September 2000)

Notes

EBM step 4: Apply the evidence

When you are satisfied that you have found the best evidence for your clinical question, either from a Cochrane systematic review, another high quality review or by critical appraisal of individual studies, the next step is to work out how the results of the search apply to your individual patient using your own clinical expertise and the values and preferences of the patient.

The questions that you should ask before you decide to apply the results of the study to your patient are:

- Is the treatment feasible in my setting?

- Is my patient so different to those in the study that the results cannot apply?

- What alternatives are available?

- Will the potential benefits of treatment outweigh the potential harms of treatment for my patient?

- What does my patient think about it?

This is sometimes called the 'external validity', or 'generalisability' of the research results.

Although this step is usually given as Step 4, which implies that it is done after Step 3 (Critical appraisal), it is entirely up to you which order you approach these two steps. For example, you will not want to waste time doing a critical appraisal of a study if it obviously will not apply in your clinical setting. On the other hand, you equally will not want to waste time working out the applicability of a study, only to find that it is a poor study. There is no easy answer to this — you will probably need to work it out on a case-by-case basis.

Steps in EBM:

1. Formulate an answerable question.

2. Track down the best evidence of outcomes available.

3. Critically appraise the evidence (ie find out how good it is).

4. Apply the evidence (integrate the results with clinical expertise and patient values).

5. Evaluate the effectiveness and efficiency of the process (to improve next time).

Is my patient similar to those in the study?

As your patients were not in the studies you have researched, you need to use your clinical expertise to decide whether they are sufficiently similar to the subjects in the studies for the results to be applicable to them. Factors that may affect your decision include:

- age (the clinical trial subjects may be older or younger than your patient)

- comorbidity (your patient may have another condition and be taking drugs that could interact with the one tested in the trial)

- compliance (you may feel that your patient is unlikely to comply with the regimen because of other factors)

- any other relevant factors.

These factors will tell you if your patient is at higher risk than the trial subjects (and likely to benefit more than seen in the trial), or at lower risk than the trial subjects (and therefore likely to benefit less).

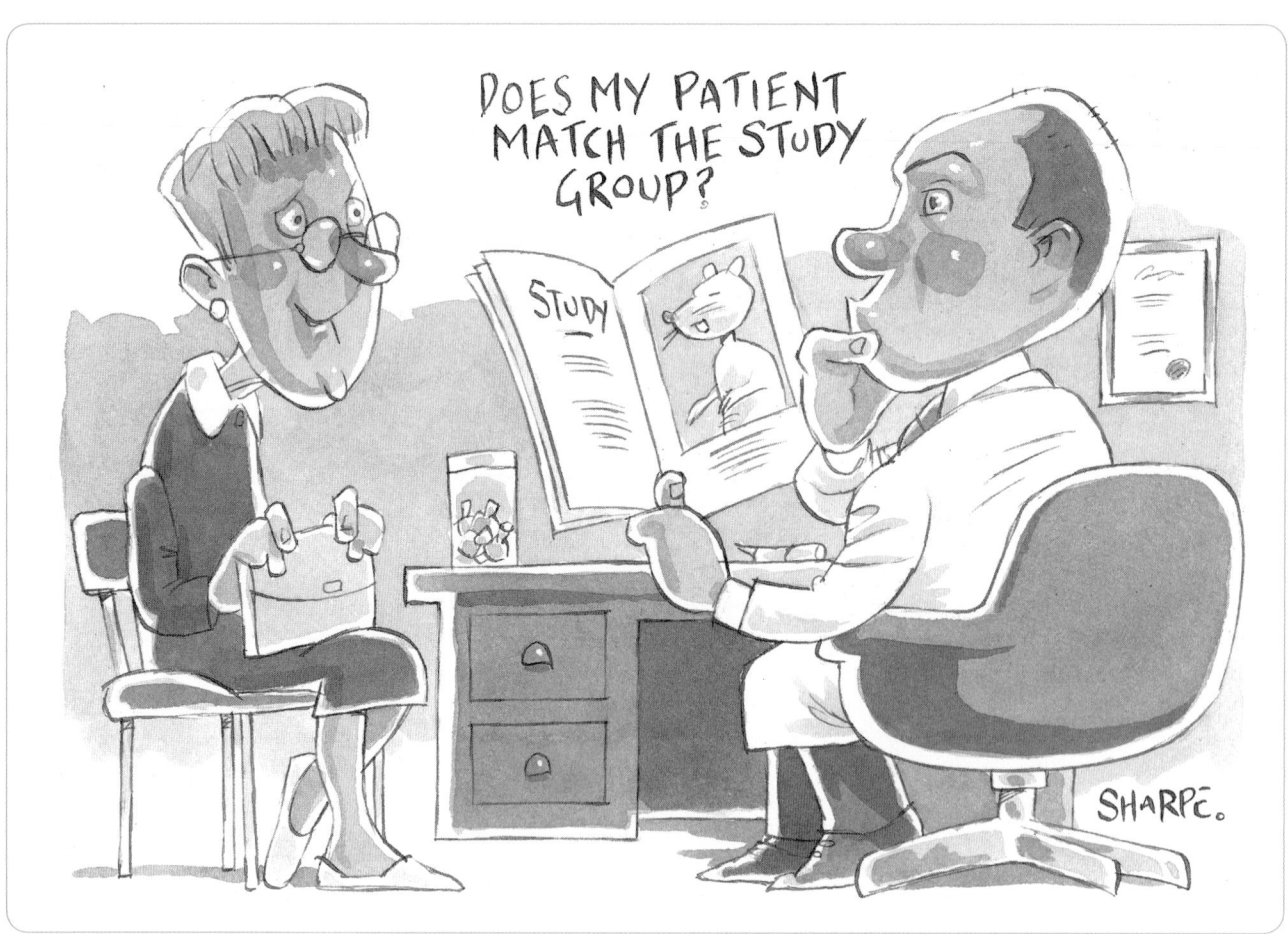

Is the treatment feasible in my setting?

You also need to assess whether the treatment, diagnostic test or other factor described in the study would be comparable in your setting. Amongst the factors that you should consider are:

- Did the study take place in a different country with different demographics?

- Did the study take place in a different clinical setting (eg general practice, hospital, emergency department)?

- Is the treatment or test available and practical in your setting?

- Can you provide the necessary monitoring and follow-up required?

- Will your patient be willing and able to comply with the treatment regimen?

What alternatives are there?

If there are other alternative treatments or procedures that you could use, then you need to weigh up which one would be most suitable for your patient, balancing the potential benefits and harms of each option. Is doing nothing an option? (This relies on your interpretation of the patient's benefits and risk of harm and what the patient thinks; see below.)

Will the potential benefits of treatment outweigh the potential harms of treatment for my patient?

If possible, from the study results, work out the number needed to treat (NNT) and, for adverse effects, the number needed to harm (NNH).

You then need to estimate your patient's risk of the outcome in question, which may be higher or lower than the control group in the study. You can then estimate the study NNT and NNH in line with your patient's personal risk factors using a method suggested by Sackett et al (2000) called the 'f method'.

The f method for estimating your patient's risk:

If your patient is twice as susceptible as those in the trial, f= 2

If your patient is half as susceptible as those in the trial, f= 0.5

Assuming the treatment produces the same relative risk reduction for patients at different levels of risk, then:

the NNT for your patient = NNT (trial)/f

Reference:

Sackett DL, Straus SE, Richardson WS et al (2000). Evidence-Based Medicine: How to Practice and Teach EBM, Churchill Livingstone, Edinburgh.

If the NNTs are similar for different treatments, look at the NNH for harmful side effects and choose the treatment with least side effects (this will also increase compliance).

What does your patient think is the best option for them?

It is important to take account of what the patient thinks, once you have explained the risks and benefits of different treatment options. The outcomes that are important to you may not be the same ones that are important to the patient, particularly where quality of life is concerned (for example, if compliance with the treatment is onerous or there are adverse effects).

Reference:

Badenoch D and Henegan C (2002). Evidence-based Medicine Toolkit, BMJ Books, London. pp37–42.

Notes

Notes

EBM step 5: Evaluate the effectiveness and efficiency of the process

It is important to keep records of your clinical questions, research results and critical appraisal of evidence, to follow up patients where you have applied the results of your searches and to record and, where appropriate, publish, outcomes. This clinical audit of your EBM activities will help you to improve what you are doing and to share your findings with colleagues. Some of the questions you may need to include in your audit are discussed below.

Are you asking any questions at all?

Ask yourself if you have managed to find the time and motivation to write down your information needs as they arise and in a way that you can follow up to a clinically useful conclusion.

If not, you may be missing some opportunities to improve your clinical performance. You could revisit the section on formulating answerable questions (EBM Step 1) and look for other strategies, such as teaming up with some colleagues to take this on as a group.

You could also try asking your colleagues 'What is the evidence for that?' whenever they make a pronouncement on the most appropriate management approach to a clinical problem.

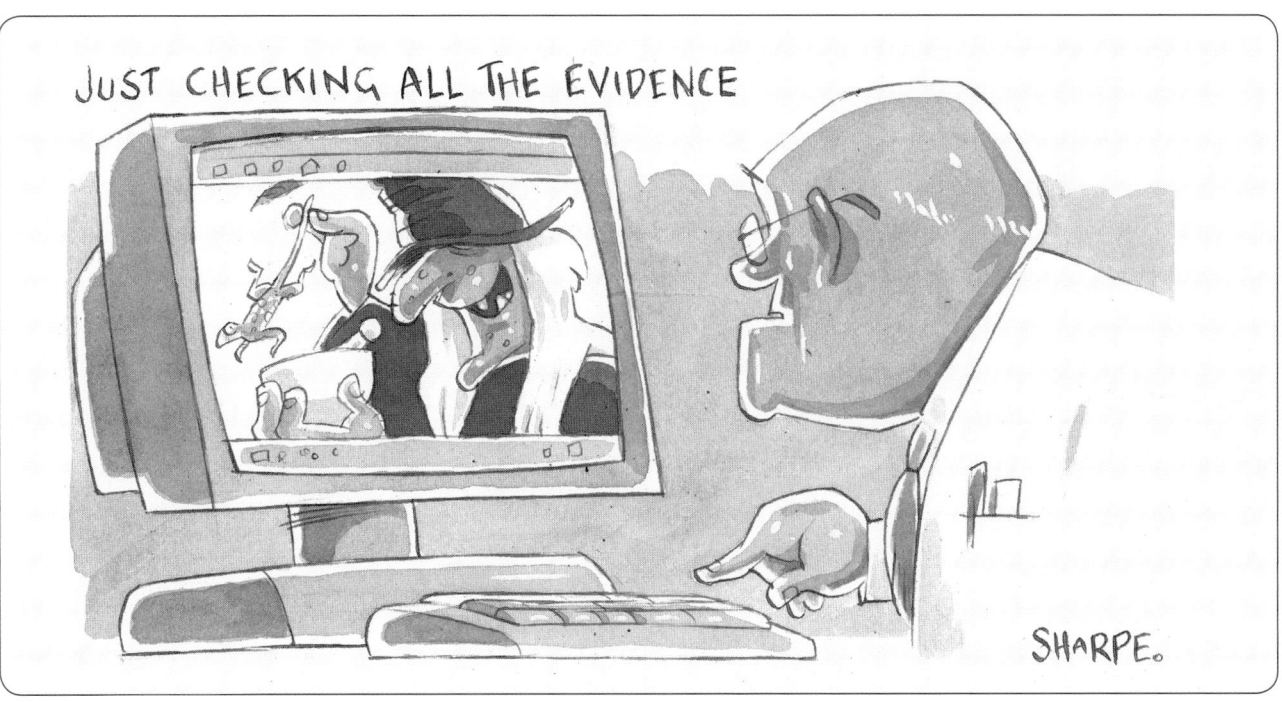

What is your success rate in asking answerable questions?

If you are generating questions, you need to ask whether your success rate in framing answerable questions is rising. If your success rate is high enough for you to keep asking questions, all is well. If you are becoming discouraged, however, you could talk to your colleagues who are having greater success and try to learn from them or attend some further professional development workshops on EBM.

How is your searching going?

If you are generating and framing answerable questions, you need to ask if you are following them up with searches and whether you have achieved access to searching hardware, sofware and the best evidence for your discipline. You could also run an audit of your questions against the resources you found most useful to find answers.

Other questions you might like to ask yourself include:

• Are you finding useful evidence from a widening array of sources?
• Are you becoming more efficient in your searching?
• Are you using MeSH headings?
• How do your searches compare to those of research librarians or other respected colleagues?

If you are having trouble with the effectiveness of your searching, you could consult your nearest health library for further information on how to access and use the available search engines and other resources.

Are you critically appraising your search results?

You should ask yourself whether you are critically appraising your evidence at all. If so, are you becoming more efficient and accurate at applying critical appraisal guidelines and measures (such as NNTs)? You may be able to find this out by comparing your results with those of colleagues who are appraising the same evidence.

Are you applying your evidence in clinical practice?

Finally, you need to ask yourself if you are integrating your critical appraisals with your clinical expertise and applying the results in your clinical practice. If so, are you becoming more accurate and efficient in adjusting some of the critical appraisal measures to fit your individual patients?

A good way to test your skills in this integration is to see whether you can use them to explain (and, hopefully, resolve) disputes about management decisions.

Reference:

Sackett DL, Strauss SE, Richardson WS et al (2000). Evidence-Based Medicine. How to practice and teach EBM, Churchill Livingstone, Edinburgh.

Notes

Notes

Part 3

Resources and further reading

Useful sources of evidence

Studies

PubMed Clinical Queries

http://www.ncbi.nlm.nih.gov/entrez/query/static/clinical.html

PubMed is a free internet MEDLINE database. The "Clinical Queries" section is a question-focused interface with filters for identifying the more appropriate studies for questions of therapy, prognosis, diagnosis, and etiology.

SUMSearch

http://sumsearch.uthscsa.edu/searchform45.htm

A super-PubMed: SUMSearch simultaneously searches multiple internet sites and collates the results. Checks for: the Merck manual, guidelines, systematic reviews, and PubMed Clinical Queries entries.

Cochrane Library & Collaboration

http://www.cochrane.org

The Cochrane Library is the single best source of reliable evidence about the effects of health care. The Cochrane Trials Registry contains over 350,000 controlled trials—the best single repository. The Cochrane Library is available free in many countries. When accessed from any internet address in these countries, it allows the option 'log on anonymously'.

CINAHL

CINAHL is the Cumulative Index to Nursing and Allied Health Literature, and is available through libraries or CKN. Unlike PubMed Clinical Queries, it has no inbuilt filters but some alternatives for CINAHL are suggested at

http://www.urmc.rochester.edu/miner/educ/ebnfilt.htm

Appraised studies

Evidence-Based Medicine

http://www.evidence-basedmedicine.com

Bi-monthly journal which summarises important recent articles from major clinical fields (family medicine, internal medicine, obstetrics and gynecology, pediatrics, psychiatry, public health, surgery). (Note: Best Evidence is the cumulated contents of ACP Journal Club (since 1991) and Evidence-Based Medicine (since 1995) in an annual CD.)

PEDro

http://www.cchs.usyd.edu.au/pedro

A physiotherapy trials database with over 2300 controlled trials, many of which have been appraised by the PEDro team at the University of Sydney.

BestBETS

http://www.bestbets.org

Provides rapid evidence-based answers to real-life clinical questions in emergency medicine, using a systematic approach to reviewing the literature. BestBETs takes into account the shortcomings of much current evidence, allowing physicians to make the best of what there is. Developed in the Emergency Department of Manchester Royal Infirmary, UK.

Syntheses

Cochrane Library and Collaboration

http://www.cochrane.org

The Cochrane Database of Systematic Reviews has over 1500 systematic reviews done by the Cochrane Collaboration. The DARE database lists other systematic reviews.

Synopses

Clinical Evidence

http://www.clinicalevidence.com

Clinical Evidence is an updated directory of evidence on the effects of clinical interventions. It summarises the current state of knowledge, ignorance and uncertainty about the prevention and treatment of clinical conditions, based on thorough searches and appraisal of the literature. It covers 20 specialties and includes 134 conditions. Updated/expanded coverage every six months in print and CD.

Bandolier

http://www.jr2.ox.ac.uk/bandolier/whatnew.html

A monthly newsletter of evidence distributed in the NHS and is freely downloadable.

TRIP Database

http://www.tripdatabase.com

Searches several different evidence-based resources including PubMed, Bandolier, and the ATTRACT question-answering service. Only allows title searches, but does allow AND, OR, NOT.

Using patient decision aids to promote evidence-based decision making

Evidence-based medicine integrates clinical experience with patients' values and the best available evidence.[1] In the past, clinicians took responsibility not only for being well informed about the benefits and harms of medical options but also for judging their value in the best interests of the patients. More recently, a shared decision making approach has been advocated in which patients are recognised as the best experts for judging values. Evidence-based decision aids are being developed and evaluated to supplement clinicians' counselling regarding values and sensitive options so that patients can understand the probable consequences of options, consider the value they place on the consequences, and participate actively with their clinician in selecting the best option for them. This editorial provides a brief overview of patient decision aids by defining them, identifying situations when they may be needed, describing their efficacy, and discussing practical issues in using them in clinical practice.

What is a patient decision aid?

Decision aids help patients to participate with their practitioners in making deliberative, personalised choices among healthcare options. The key elements of decision aids have been described by the Cochrane Collaboration[2] as

INFORMATION TAILORED TO THE PATIENT'S HEALTH STATUS

Information is provided on the condition, disease, or developmental transition stimulating the decision; the healthcare options available; the outcomes of options, including how they affect patient functioning; and the probabilities associated with outcomes.

VALUES CLASSIFICATION

Values clarification exercises are used to explicitly consider and communicate the personal importance of each benefit or harm by using such strategies as balance scales, relevance charts, or trade off techniques.

EXAMPLES OF OTHER PATIENTS

Patients often like to learn from others who have faced the same situation, and aids can give a balanced illustration of how others deliberate about options and arrive at decisions based on their personal situation.

GUIDANCE OR COACHING IN SHARED DECISION MAKING

Skills and confidence in participating in decision making are developed by guiding patients in the steps involved and by discussing values and personal issues.

MEDIUM OF DELIVERY

Decision aids are delivered as self administered tools or practitioner administered tools in one to one or group sessions.

Possible media include decision boards, interactive videodiscs, personal computers, audiotapes, audio guided workbooks, and pamphlets.

This definition clearly shows that information is a necessary but not an exclusive element of decision aids. People need to learn how to personalise this information and how to communicate their personal issues and values to their practitioners. Decision aids are meant to supplement rather than to replace counselling, and follow up with a practitioner is a necessary part of providing decision support.

The Cochrane Collaboration also defines what decision aids are not.[2] They do not include educational materials that inform people about health issues in general ways but that do not support decision making about a specific set of options relevant to the patient. Decision aids are not passive informed consent materials in which a clinician recommends a strategy and then provides information for providing consent. And finally, they are not interventions designed to promote compliance with a recommended option rather than a choice based on personal values.

When do you need a decision aid?

The use of decision aids is usually reserved for circumstances in which patients need to carefully deliberate about the personal value of the benefits and harms of options. Clinicians are beginning to get easy access to high quality summaries of the benefits and harms of management options in such evidence-based resources as *Clinical Evidence*.[3] Kassirer[4] lists some indications for explicitly eliciting patients' values in clinical practice, including situations where:

- Options have major differences in outcomes or complications
- Decisions require making tradeoffs between short term and long term outcomes
- One choice can result in a small chance of a grave outcome
- There are marginal differences in outcomes between options.

Patient characteristics may also determine the need for a decision aid. For example, if patients are risk averse or if they attach unusual importance to certain possible outcomes (eg, risks for disease from blood transfusions), a decision aid might be helpful.

Another useful strategy for determining the need for a decision aid is to classify treatment policies as standards, guidelines, or options by using Eddy's definitions.[5] For standards of care in which outcomes are known and patients' preferences are generally consistent in favouring an intervention, decision aids may be less useful and conventional informed consent procedures more appropriate. Examples include the use of insulin in patients with type I diabetes mellitus or the use of antibiotics in patients with an infection known to be responsive to antibiotics.

List of Decision Aids

Condition specific decision aids	Delivery format	Publication
Breast cancer surgery	Audio cassette/booklet	*Health Expectations* 1998;**1**:23–36
		Med Decis Making 2001;**21**:1–6
Atrial fibrillation and antithrombotic treatment	Audio cassette/booklet	*JAMA* 1999;**282**:737–43
		J Gen Intern Med 2000;**15**:723–30
Cardiac ischaemic treatment	Video disc	*Health Expectations* 1998;**1**:50–61
		J Gen Intern Med 2000;**15**:685–93
		J Gen Intern Med 1996;**11**:373–6
Menopause options	Audio cassette/booklet	*Patient Educ Counsel* 1998;**33**:267–79
		Med Decis Making 1998;**18**:295–303
Benign prostatic hyperplasia treatment	Video/video disc	*Dis Management Clinical Outcomes* 1997;**1**:5–14
		Med Care 1995;**33**:765–70
Prostate specific antigen testing	Video cassette/booklet	*J Gen Intern Med* 1996;**11**:342–9
		Arch Fam Med 1999;**8**:333–40

In contrast, when a treatment policy is classified as a guideline or an option, decision aids may be indicated because outcomes may be less certain or values for the benefits relative to the harms are more variable or unknown. For example, good evidence exists that amniocentesis performed on pregnant women who are >35 years of age is effective in detecting abnormalities, but not all women choose the procedure because their values about the medical options and potential outcomes differ. Benign prostatic hypertrophy is another example because it has several management options (watchful waiting, drugs, or surgery) and potential outcomes (amount of symptom relief *v* drug side effects or surgical risks of incontinence and impotence) that each patient may value differently.

Do decision aids work?

Evaluation studies from a Cochrane systematic overview of trials[2] and 2 general reviews[6 7] have shown that decision aids improve decision making by:

- Reducing the proportion of patients who are uncertain about what to choose
- Increasing patients' knowledge of the problem, options, and outcomes
- Creating realistic personal expectations (perceived probabilities) of outcomes
- Improving the agreement between choices and a patients' values
- Reducing some elements of decisional conflict (feeling uncertain, uninformed, unclear about values, and unsupported in decision making)
- Increasing participation in decision making without adversely affecting anxiety.

However, the impact of decision aids on satisfaction with decision making is more uncertain. More research is needed on the clinical, behavioural, and service utilisation outcomes of decisions. We also need to know which decision aids work best with which decisions and which types of patients and how acceptable decision aids are to practitioners and to diverse groups and cultures.

Questions also exist about the essential elements in decision aids. Although decision aids have been quite beneficial relative to usual care, the differences between simpler and more detailed aids have often been marginal.

How do you know a particular decision aid is a good one?

The definition of a patient decision aid is open to broad interpretation, and materials of variable quality have been produced. Consumers expect to receive free health information and may have difficulty distinguishing the wheat from the "free" chaff unless certain standards are set in their development.

A high quality decision aid should

- Be evidence-based, using evidence-based statements of benefits and risks from credible sources; refer to the quality and consistency of empirical studies; and use systematic overviews that extend shelf life and enhance updating
- Be balanced in presenting all options (including doing nothing), the benefits and risks of all options, and (when available) examples of others' decisions and opinions
- Have credible developers with expertise as evidence interpreters, communicators, practitioners, consumers, and disseminators
- Be up to date by using expiry dates indicating the expected shelf life of the information, mentioning upcoming trials that may shift policy, and demonstrating linkage to an ongoing and credible evidence analysis process (eg, the International Cochrane overview groups, the US Agency for Health Care Research and Quality evidence centres, and the Canadian Cancer Care Ontario Practice Guidelines Initiative)
- Identify conflicts of interests of developers and funding sources
- Provide evidence of evaluation describing how the aid improves decision making.

HOW DO YOU ACCESS THESE DECISION AIDS?

The Cochrane decision aids review group is assembling a list of all decision aids available and under evaluation. Most aids have been used in research environments for evaluation. The table lists the decision aids that have been developed, evaluated, and made available to others. (For a complete list of decision aids that have been developed, please see http://www.ohri.ca/programs/clinical-epidemiology/ohdec.)

Many of the decision aids are self administered in video, computer, or audio guided workbook formats so that they can be used feasibly in settings with limited personnel and limited time for counselling. Therefore, the time that practitioners can spend on counselling focuses on personal deliberation rather than providing factual information. Some larger health services (eg, health maintenance organisations in the US) also employ telephone health coaches: patients are referred to them to access materials and to ask questions in preparation for follow up counselling with their individual practitioners. This delivery strategy may become more feasible in other countries as tele-health services expand (eg, NHS Direct in the UK and InfoSante in Quebec, Canada).

Because of the amount of time required to make "from scratch" evidence based decisions, evidence based practitioners will often not succeed in reviewing the original literature that bears on a clinical dilemma they face. Thus, two reasons exist why training evidence based practitioners will not, alone, achieve evidence based practice. Firstly, many clinicians will not be interested in gaining a high level of sophistication in using the original literature, and, secondly, those who do will often be short of time in applying these skills.

In our residency programme we have observed that even trainees who are less interested in evidence based methods develop a respect for, and ability to track down and use, secondary sources of preappraised evidence (evidence based resources) that provide immediately applicable conclusions. Having mastered this restricted set of skills, these trainees (whom we call evidence users) can become highly competent, up to date practitioners who deliver evidence based care. Time limitations dictate that evidence based practitioners also rely heavily on conclusions from preappraised resources. Such resources, which apply a methodological filter to original investigations and therefore ensure a minimal standard of validity, include the *Cochrane Library, ACP Journal Club, Evidence-based Medicine*, and *Best Evidence* and an increasing number of computer decision support systems. Thus, producing more comprehensive and more easily accessible preappraised resources is a second strategy for ensuring evidence based care.

The availability of evidence based resources and recommendations will still be insufficient to produce consistent evidence based care. Habit, local practice patterns, and product marketing may often be stronger determinants of practice. Controlled trials have shown that traditional continuing education has little effect on combating these forces and changing doctors' behaviour.[4] On the other hand, approaches that do change targeted clinical behaviours include one to one conversations with an expert, computerised alerts and reminders, preceptorships, advice from opinion leaders, and targeted audit and feedback.[5-7] Other effective strategies include restricted drug formularies, financial incentives, and institutional guidelines. Application of these strategies, which do not demand even a rudimentary ability to use the original medical literature and instead focus on behaviour change, thus constitute a third strategy for achieving evidence based care.

Nevertheless, there remain reasons for ensuring that medical trainees achieve the highest possible skill level in evidence based practice. Firstly, attempts to change doctors' practice will sometimes be directed to ends other than evidence based care, such as increasing specific drug use or reducing healthcare costs. Clinicians with advanced skills in interpreting the medical literature will be able to determine the extent to which these attempts are consistent with the best evidence. Secondly, they will be able to use the original literature when preappraised synopses and evidence based recommendations are unavailable. At the same time, educators, managers, and policymakers should be aware that the widespread availability of comprehensive preappraised evidence based summaries and the implementation of strategies known to change clinicians' behaviour will both be necessary to ensure high levels of evidence based health care.

Gordon H Guyatt
Maureen O Meade
Roman Z Jaeschke
Deborah J Cook
R Brian Haynes *clinical epidemiologists*

Department of Clinical Epidemiology and Biostatistics, McMaster University, Hamilton, Ontario, Canada L8N 3Z5
(guyatt@fhs.csu.mcmaster.ca)

We thank the following for their input: Eric Bass, Pat Brill-Edwards, Antonio Dans, Paul Glasziou, Lee Green, Anne Holbrook, Hui Lee, Tom Newman, Andrew Oxman, and Jack Sinclair

1   Evidence-based Medicine Working Group. Evidence-based medicine: a new approach to teaching the practice of medicine. *JAMA* 1992;268:2420-5.
2   Sackett DL, Richardson WS, Rosenberg W, Haynes RB. *Evidence-based medicine: how to practice and teach EBM.* London: Churchill Livingstone, 1997:12-6.
3   McColl A, Smith H, White P, Field J. General practitioners' perceptions of the route to evidence based medicine: a questionnaire survey. *BMJ* 1998;316:361-5.
4   Davis DA, Thomson MA, Oxman AD, Haynes RB. Changing physician performance. *JAMA* 1995;274:700-5.
5   Oxman AD, Thomson MA, Davis DA, Haynes RB. No magic bullets: a systematic review of 102 trials of interventions to improve professional practice. *Can Med Assoc J* 1995;153:1423-31.
6   Grimshaw JM, Russell IT. Achieving health gain through clinical guidelines II: Ensuring guidelines change medical practice. *Quality in Health Care* 1994;3:45-52.
7   Hunt DL, Haynes RB, Hanna SE, Smith K. Effects of computer-based clinical decision support systems on physician behaviour and patient outcomes: a systematic review. *JAMA* 1998;280:1339-46.

Systems for emergency care

Integrating the components is the challenge

The British government's announcement of the first 36 new NHS "walk in centres" is the latest in a series of important changes in the provision of immediate access services over the past 20 years.[1] A study of first contact out of hours care in England 16 years ago recorded only attendances at accident and emergency departments, general practitioners' home visits and telephone advice, and visits by deputising services.[2] Contacts with regional trauma centres, minor injury units, general practitioners' out of hours cooperative treatment centres, community pharmacies, and community mental health teams, for example, were either negligible or non-existent.

The recent development of triage and advice telephone services, such as NHS Direct,[3] has further complicated the picture, and now the government proposes 36 walk in centres (with more under consideration) to "offer a service to the public, when the public need it and where the public need it."[1] These services, based in shops, health centres, and hospitals will be nurse led, with access to general practitioners in some cases, and will offer extended opening hours, including

BMJ 2000;320:955-6

influence public health policies and priorities; link their name to prestigious non-governmental organisations, United Nations agencies, and doctors; affect the direction and outcome of research; create dependency; create public confusion about the real causes of poverty.

Of course they have a responsibility to research and improve products, and of necessity they must employ scientists. But such involvement inevitably creates a conflict of interest, and this is why corporations go to such lengths to ensure that their scientists sit on influential committees such as the Committee on Medical Aspects of Food, Codex Alimentarius Commission (the commission that produces recommended food standards for the world), the new Food Standards Agency, or the European Scientific Committee for Food. Some of these committees have already had an important influence on food laws and the public and are part of the reason that UK law is so weak and that so few women in Britain breast feed. Surely the public should be able to trust that such public bodies do not favour commercial interests over public health.

As long ago as 1983, Professor John Reid of the University of Cape Town said to industry representatives at the 12th annual meeting of the World Sugar Research Organisation: "There is a hidden agenda in the research support business. Those who accept your [industries'] support are often perceived to be less likely to give you a bad scientific press. They may come up with the results that cause you problems, but they will put them in a context in a way that leaves you happier than had they emanated from someone not receiving your support. My own observation and comment is that this hidden effect is powerful, more powerful certainly than we care to state loudly, from the point of view of honour either in science or in industry. It takes a lot to bite the hand that feeds you."

The world is facing many difficult problems that need the close attention of everyone concerned with public health. If sustainable solutions are to be found, surely it is imperative that adequate public funds are set aside for this purpose—instead of money that has already been allocated by industry for an entirely different purpose, namely marketing.

1 Mehdi T, Wagner-Rizvi T. *Feeding fiasco—pushing commercial infant foods in Pakistan.* Islamabad: Network for the Rational Use of Medication, 1998. (Available from Baby Milk Action.)
2 Sokol E, Thiagarajah S, Allain A. *Breaking the rules, stretching the rules.* Penang: International Baby Food Action Network, 1998. (Available from Baby Milk Action.)
3 Taylor A. Violations of the international code of marketing of breast milk substitutes: prevalence in four countries. *BMJ* 1998;316:1117-22.

Getting research findings into practice
Using research findings in clinical practice

S E Straus, D L Sackett

In clinical practice caring for patients generates many questions about diagnosis, prognosis, and treatment that challenge health professionals to keep up to date with the medical literature. A study of general practitioners in North America found that two clinically important questions arose for every three patients seen.[1] The challenge in keeping abreast of the medical literature is the volume of literature. General physicians who want to keep up with relevant journals face the task of examining 19 articles a day 365 days a year.[2]

One approach to meeting these challenges and avoiding clinical entropy is to learn how to practise evidence based medicine. Evidence based medicine involves integrating clinical expertise with the best available clinical evidence derived from systematic research.[3] Individual clinical expertise is the proficiency and judgment that each clinician acquires through clinical experience and practice. Best available clinical evidence is clinically relevant research which may be from the basic sciences of medicine, but especially that derived from clinical research that is patient centred, that evaluates the accuracy and precision of diagnostic tests and prognostic markers, and the efficacy and safety of therapeutic, rehabilitative, and preventive regimens. This paper focuses on what evidence based medicine is and how it can be practised by busy clinicians.

Summary points

Practising evidence based medicine allows clinicians to keep up with the rapidly growing body of medical literature

Evidence based medicine improves clinicians' skills in asking answerable questions and finding the best evidence to answer these questions

Evidence based medicine can provide a framework for critically appraising evidence

Practising evidence based medicine encourages clinicians to integrate valid and useful evidence with clinical expertise and each patient's unique features, and enables clinicians to apply evidence to the treatment of patients

The practice of evidence based medicine is a process of lifelong self directed learning in which caring for patients creates a need for clinically important information about diagnoses, prognoses, treatment, and other healthcare issues. The box at the bottom of the next page illustrates the five steps necessary to the practice of evidence based medicine.

This is the fifth in a series of eight articles analysing the gap between research and practice

NHS Research and Development Centre for Evidence Based Medicine, Nuffield Department of Clinical Medicine, Oxford Radcliffe Hospital NHS Trust, Oxford OX3 9DU
S E Straus, *deputy director*
D L Sackett, *director*

Correspondence to: Dr Straus sharon.straus@ clinical-medicine.ox.ac.uk

Series editors: Andrew Haines and Anna Donald

BMJ 1998;317:339-42

Asking answerable clinical questions

Formulating clear, focused clinical questions is a prerequisite to answering them. Four components of the question must be specified: the patient or problem being addressed; the intervention being considered (a cause, prognostic factor, or treatment); another intervention for comparison, when relevant; and the clinical outcomes of interest.[4] The intervention could be from a clinical trial (for example, a drug) or from nature (for example, sex or age).

To illustrate how many questions may arise in the treatment of one patient consider a 65 year old man with a history of cirrhosis and ascites secondary to alcohol abuse who presents to accident and emergency with haematemesis. The patient is taking a diuretic. On examination he is disoriented and looks unwell but is afebrile. His blood pressure is 90/60 supine and 70/50 while seated; his heart rate is 100 beats per minute while supine. In addition to spider naevi and gynaeco-mastia he has ascites. Bowel sounds are present.

Dozens of questions may arise in treating this patient; some are summarised in the box opposite. The questions cover a wide spectrum: clinical findings, aetiology, differential diagnosis, diagnostic tests, prognosis, treatment, prevention, and self improvement.[4] Given their breadth and number, and knowing that clinicians are likely to have only about 30 minutes in a week to address any of them,[5] it is necessary to pare the questions down to just one. This can be done by considering the question that would be most important to the patient's wellbeing and balancing it against a number of factors including which question appears most feasible to answer, which question is most interesting to the clinician, and which question is most likely to be raised in subsequent patients and could provide information for them. For this patient the question becomes: in a patient with cirrhosis and suspected variceal bleeding does treatment with soma-tostatin decrease the risk of death?

Searching for the best evidence

A focused question sharpens the search for the best evidence. Strategies that increase the sensitivity and specificity of searches have been developed and are available both in paper[4] and electronic forms (for example, at the site established by the NHS Research and Development Centre for Evidence-Based Medi-

---

Questions to be asked in treating patient with cirrhosis and haematemesis

Clinical findings
Which is the most accurate way of diagnosing ascites on physical examination: fluid wave or shifting dullness?

Aetiology
Can gastrointestinal bleeding cause confusion in a patient with cirrhosis and ascites?

Differential diagnosis
In a patient with cirrhosis and ascites which is most likely to cause gastrointestinal bleeding, variceal haemorrhage or peptic ulcer disease?

Diagnostic tests
In a patient with suspected alcohol abuse is the use of the CAGE questionnaire specific for diagnosing alcohol abuse?[6]

Prognosis
Does gastrointestinal bleeding increase the risk of death in a patient with cirrhosis?

Treatment
Does treatment with somatostatin decrease the risk of death in a patient with cirrhosis and variceal bleeding?

Prevention
Does treatment with a β blocker decrease the risk of morbidity and mortality in a patient with cirrhosis, ascites, and varices?

Self improvement
To improve my understanding of the pathophysiology of ascites would I gain more from spending an hour in the library reading a textbook or spending 15 minutes on the ward computer looking at the CD ROM version of the same textbook?

---

cine at URL: http://cebm.jr2.ox.ac.uk). Librarians also may be helpful in guiding and assisting searches.

The types and number of resources are rapidly expanding and some of them have already undergone critical appraisal during development. Most rigorous of these are the systematic reviews on the effects of health care that have been generated by the Cochrane Collaboration, readily available as *The Cochrane Library* on compact disc,[7] and accompanied by abstracts for critically appraised overviews in the *Database of Abstracts of Reviews of Effectiveness* created by the NHS Centre for Reviews and Dissemination.[7] A systematic review from *The Cochrane Library* is exhaustive and therefore takes years to generate; reviews from the *Database of Abstracts of Reviews of Effectiveness* can be generated in months. Still faster is the appearance of clinical articles about diagnosis, prognosis, treatment, quality of care, and economics that pass both specific methodological standards (so that their results are likely to be valid) and clinical scrutiny for relevance and that appear in evidence based journals such as the *ACP Journal Club, Evidence-Based Medicine,* and *Evidence-Based Cardiovascular Medicine.* This selection process reduces the amount of clinical literature by 98% to the 2% that is most methodologically rigorous and useful to clinician.[8] In these journals, the evidence is summa-rised in structured abstracts and a clinical expert adds commentary to the article which allows the reader to place the findings in context.

An electronic publication, *Best Evidence,* combines the contents of the *ACP Journal Club* with the contents

---

Steps necessary in practising evidence based medicine

• Convert the need for information into clinically relevant, answerable questions

• Find, in the most efficient way, the best evidence with which to answer these questions (whether this evidence comes from clinical examination, laboratory tests, published research, or other sources)

• Critically appraise the evidence for its validity (closeness to the truth) and usefulness (clinical applicability)

• Integrate the appraisal with clinical expertise and apply the results to clinical practice

• Evaluate your performance

---

of *Evidence-Based Medicine* in an easily searched compact disc.[9] In caring for the patient with cirrhosis and gastrointestinal bleeding a search of *The Cochrane Library* using the term "variceal bleed" identified the Cochrane review that evaluated the use of somatostatin versus placebo or no treatment in acute bleeding oesophageal varices.[10]

Some evidence based materials also appear on the internet, including those of the Cochrane Collaboration (URL: http://hiru.mcmaster.ca/COCHRANE) and some sites include clinically useful evidence about diagnosis, prognosis, and treatment. For example, the site established by the NHS Research and Development Centre for Evidence-Based Medicine (URL given above) permits browsers to apply the specificity of shifting dullness and the sensitivity of a history of ankle swelling to diagnose patients thought to have ascites; this information could be used to answer some of the questions posed in the diagnosis of the patient with cirrhosis. If the foregoing strategies for gaining rapid access to evidence based medicine fail clinicians can resort to the time honoured and increasingly user friendly systems for accessing the current literature via Medline and Embase, employing methodological quality filters to maximise the yield of high quality evidence.

Critically appraising the evidence

Once clinicians find potentially useful evidence it has to be critically appraised and its validity and usefulness determined. Guidelines have been generated to help clinicians evaluate the validity of evidence about diagnostic tests (was there an independent, blind comparison with a gold standard of diagnosis?), treatment (was the assignment of patients to treatments really randomised?), prognostic markers (was an appropriate sample of patients assembled at a uniform point in their illness?), and clinical guidelines or other strategies for improving the quality of care.[4 11] Worksheets for applying guidelines to determine whether findings are valid are also available (see the address of the NHS Research and Development site given above). The trend towards publishing more informative abstracts also makes it easier for clinicians to determine whether research findings are applicable to their patients.

For the patient with cirrhosis and haematemesis, an assessment of the Cochrane review finds that it is valid, and the results showed that somatostatin did not have a statistically significant effect on survival. The confidence interval for the effect on mortality was wide, suggesting that larger studies need to be done to find definitive answers.[9]

After finding an article and determining if its results are valid and useful, it is often helpful to file a summary so that it can be referred to again or passed along to colleagues. One way to do this is to prepare a one page summary that includes information on the patient, the evidence, and the clinical bottom line organised as a critically appraised topic (CAT).[12] CATmakers (for constructing, storing, and printing information on critically appraised topics, and for calculating likelihood ratios and numbers needed to treat) are becoming more widely available, as are websites where they can be stored or retrieved (see the NHS site described earlier). Information on critically appraised topics are more useful to those who produce them

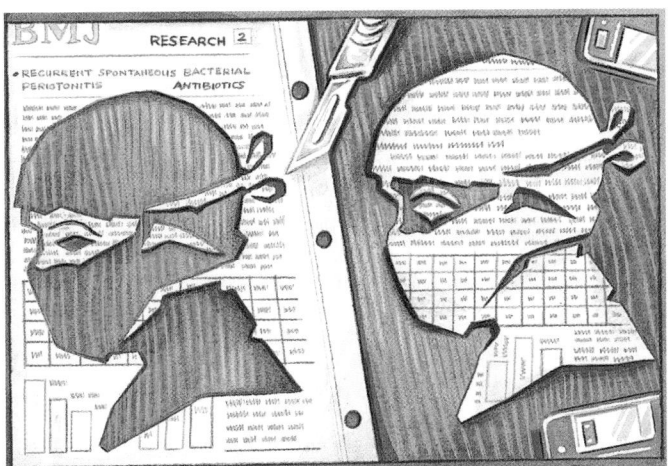

(clinicians who produce them become more effective in searching and critically appraising evidence) than to potential users (since the summaries undergo little peer review and may be useful mainly for their citations).

Applying the evidence

Applying the results of critical appraisals involves the essential second element of evidence based medicine: integrating the evidence with clinical expertise and knowledge of the unique features of patients and their situations, rights, and expectations. Only after these things have been considered can we then decide whether and how to incorporate the evidence into the care of a particular patient. In the case of the patient with cirrhosis and haematemesis, there was insufficient power in the review to determine if the risk of mortality would be reduced with the use of somatostatin. The study did report that one unit of blood was saved in treating each patient, but this is unlikely to be considered cost effective. Another factor to consider is whether endoscopic services are available for sclerotherapy or ligation of varices, and if somatostatin should be used in the interim if endoscopy is not readily available. Accordingly, the decision of whether to treat the patient with somatostatin would have to grow out of a therapeutic alliance with the patient who would have to be informed about the potential risks and benefits of this treatment.

Evaluating your performance

To complete the cycle of practising evidence based medicine clinicians should evaluate their own performance. Clinicians can evaluate their progress at each stage by asking whether their questions were answerable, by asking if good evidence was found quickly, by asking if evidence was effectively appraised, and by asking whether the integration of the appraisal with clinical expertise and the patient's unique features left them with a rational, acceptable management strategy. This fifth step of self evaluation allows clinicians to focus on earlier steps that may need improvement in the future. For example, for the patient with cirrhosis and haematemesis we can assess the application of the evidence about the treatment of variceal bleeding and determine whether we discussed the risks and benefits of treatment with the patient and whether the patient's own values were incorporated into our discussion.

Conclusions

Can medical practice be evidence based? Recent audits have been encouraging; a general medicine service at a district general hospital affiliated with a university found that 53% of patients admitted to the service received primary treatments that had been validated in randomised controlled trials or systematic reviews of randomised controlled trials; an additional 29% of patients received care based on convincing non-experimental evidence.[13] Three quarters of all of the evidence had been immediately available in the form of critically appraised topic summaries, and the remaining quarter was identified and applied by asking answerable questions at the time of admission, rapidly finding good evidence, quickly determining its validity and usefulness, swiftly integrating it with clinical expertise and each patient's unique features, and offering it to the patients. Similar results have been found in a study performed at a psychiatric hospital,[14] general practitioners' office,[15] and a paediatric surgery department.[16]

Practising evidence based medicine is one way for clinicians to keep up to date with the exponential growth in medical literature, not just by more efficient browsing but by improving our skills in asking questions, finding the best evidence, critically appraising it, integrating it with our clinical expertise and our patients' unique features, and applying the results to clinical practice. When added to conscientiously practised clinical skills and constantly developing clinical expertise, sound external evidence can be applied efficiently and effectively to our patients' problems.

Funding: SES is supported by the R Samuel McLaughlin Foundation.

Conflict of interest: None.

The articles in this series are adapted from Getting research findings into practice, edited by Andrew Haines and Anna Donald, and published by BMJ Books.

1 Covell DG, Uman GC, Manning PR. Information needs in office practice: are they being met? *Ann Intern Med* 1985;103:596-9.
2 Davidoff F, Haynes RB, Sackett DL, Smith R. Evidence-based medicine: a new journal to help doctors identify the information they need. *BMJ* 1995;310:1085-6.
3 Sackett DL, Rosenberg WMC, Gray JAM, Richardson WS. Evidence based medicine: what it is and what it isn't. *BMJ* 1996;312:71-2.
4 Sackett DL, Richardson WS, Rosenberg WMC, Haynes RB. *Evidence-based medicine: how to practice and teach EBM*. London: Churchill Livingstone, 1997.
5 Sackett DL. Using evidence-based medicine to help physicians keep up-to-date. *Serials* 1996;9:178-81.
6 Bush B, Shaw S, Cleary P, Delbanco TL, Aronson MD. Screening for alcohol abuse using the CAGE questionnaire. *Am J Med* 1987;82:231-5.
7 *The Cochrane Library* [database on disk and CD ROM]. Cochrane Collaboration. Oxford: Update Software; 1998. Updated quarterly.
8 Sackett DL, Haynes RB. 13 steps, 100 people, 1 000 000 thanks. *Evidence Based Med* 1997;2:101-2.
9 *Best Evidence* [database on CD ROM]. Philadelphia: American College of Physicians, 1996.
10 Gotzsche PC. Somatostatin or octreotide vs placebo or no treatment in acute bleeding oesophageal varices. In: Gluud C, Jorgenson T, Koretz RL, Morabito A, Pagliaro L, Poyunard T et al, eds. Hepato-biliary module, Cochrane Database of Systematic Reviews [updated 23 April 1997]. *The Cochrane Library*. Cochrane Collaboration; Issue 2. Oxford: Update Software; 1998. Updated quarterly.
11 Oxman AD, Sackett DL, Guyatt GH for the Evidence-based medicine working group. How to get started. *JAMA* 1993;270:2093-5.
12 Sauve JS, Lee HM, Farkouh ME, Sackett DL. The critically appraised topic: a practical approach to learning critical appraisal. *Ann R Coll Physicians Surg Canada* 1995;28:396-8.
13 Ellis J. Mulligan I, Rower J, Sackett DL. Inpatient general medicine is evidence based. *Lancet* 1995;346:407-10.
14 Geddes JR, Game D, Jenkins NE, Peterson LA, Pottinger GR, Sackett DL. What proportion of primary psychiatric interventions are based on randomised evidence? *Qual Health Care* 1996;5:215-7.
15 Gill P, Dowell AC, Neal RP, Smith N, Heywood P, Wilson AK. Evidence based general practice: a retrospective study of interventions in our training practice. *BMJ* 1996;312:819-21.
16 Kenny SE, Shankar KR, Rentala R, Lamont GL, Lloyd DA. Evidence-based surgery: interventions in a regional paediatric surgical unit. *Arch Dis Child* 1997;76:50-3.

A memorable patient
Happy ending

She had been admitted that Saturday morning as an "acute abdomen," but the surgical registrar could not make a diagnosis and passed her over to the paediatricians. My senior house officer emphasised her concerns with her first sentence to me over the telephone: "If you don't see her she'll die."

The girl was almost 4 years old, quiet, and toxic. Severe abdominal pain and vomiting continued. The abdomen was scaphoid and not significantly tender. X ray examinations were unhelpful. The diagnosis was obscure, but it was clear that necrosis was setting in and we persuaded the surgeons that the abdomen should be opened.

There had been a massive herniation of the malrotated small bowel through a hole in the peritoneum. Once released the circulation seemed to recover and the surgical registrar closed up after some 40 minutes. She improved but 18 hours later she collapsed in severe pain and peripheral circulatory failure.

I sought advice from Professor (now Sir) Christopher Booth, who gave me the names of surgeons who practised interval resection for patients with mesenteric thrombosis. By Sunday morning I had gathered sufficient evidence of the success of such management, via long distance telephone calls, to be able to persuade the consultant to resect as much as necessary. He agreed "so long as the parents do not blame the surgeon if she dies on the table." "They'll blame you if you don't even try," I thought. Out came 10 feet of gangrenous bowel. She was left with only six inches of jejunum and seven of ileum but, critically, all the duodenum and colon and the ileocaecal valve.

She immediately looked better and back on the ward we fed her on solid food from the fourth day. After many weeks we sent her home still vomiting. Her mother, despite six other siblings to look after, was, I felt, better able than the ward to feed and refeed her as often as she needed.

She came to outpatients regularly and gained no weight for five months. Very weak, she was carried everywhere, but then one day I heard her little footsteps as well as her parents' approaching the consulting room door. I knew that she was better before I saw her. She had gained two pounds. The only supplements were children's multivitamins and extra vitamin D—no folate and no B12. She did not need them. She did need a low fat diet (over which we compromised in order to maintain her appetite) and some iron later in her teens. The retroperistalsis subsided and the remaining bowel grew and its mucosa hypertrophied, but as a girl she refused any further investigation so I could not study this recovery.

She grew into a slender, beautiful, and otherwise healthy young lady. I went to her wedding. She is now 37, has three lovely children, all breast fed after appropriately supplemented pregnancies. She is fully active and a recent health check found "nothing to cause concern and more bowel than the doctor had expected."

Her healthy survival has much to do with the plentiful provision of solid food in the early days and her parents' dedication.

Patricia Mortimer, retired paediatrician, Enfield

25 Gaube J, Feucht HH, Laufs R, Polywka S, Fingscheidt E, Müller HE. Hepatitis A, B und C als desmoterische Infektionen. *Gesundheitswesen* 1993;55:246-29.
26 Vlahov D, Nelson KE, Quinn TC, Kending N. Prevalence and incidence of hepatitis C virus infection among male prison inmates in Maryland. *Eur J Epidemiol* 1993;9:566-9.
27 Crofts N, Steward T, Hearne P, Xin YP, Breschkin AM, Locarnini SA. Spread of bloodborne viruses among Australian prison entrants. *BMJ* 1995;310:285-8.
28 Anon C, del Olmo JA, Llovet F, Serra MA, Gilabert S, Rodriguez F, et al. Virus C de la hepatitis entre la poblacion penitenciaria de Valencia. *Rev Esp Enferm Dig* 1995;87:505-8.
29 Ford PM, White C, Kaufmann H, MacTavish J, Pearson M, Ford S, et al. Voluntary anonymous linked study of the prevalence of HIV infection and hepatitis C among inmates in a Canadian federal penitentiary for women. *Can Med Assoc J* 1995;153:1605-9.
30 Polych C, Sabo D. Gender politics, pain, and illness. The AIDS epidemic in North American prisons. In: Sabo DF, Gordon F, eds. *Men's health and illness.* Thousand Oaks, CA: Sage, 1995:139-57.

31 Nelles J, Fuhrer A. Drug and HIV prevention at the Hindelbank penitentiary. Abridged report of the evaluation results. Mandated by the Swiss Federal Office of Public Health, Bern 1995. (Also available in German and French.)
32 Nelles J, Fuhrer A, eds. *Harm reduction in prison. Strategies against drugs, AIDS and risk behaviour.* Bern: Lang, 1997.
33 Nelles J, Fuhrer A. *Kurzevaluation des Pilotprojekts Drogen- und Aidspräventtion in den Basler Gefängnissen.* Bern: Bundesamtes für Gesundheit, 1997.
34 Pape U, Böttger A, Pfeiffer C. Wissenschaftliche Begleitung und Beurteilung des geplanten Spritzentauschprogramms im Rahmen eines Modellversuchs der Justizbehörde der Freien Hansestadt Hamburg. Konzeption eines empirischen Forschungsprojekts. Hannover: Kriminologisches Forschungsinstitut Niedersachsen, 1996. (Forschungsbericht Nr 54.)
35 Meyenberg R, Stöver H, Jacob J, Pospeschill M. Infektionsprophylaxe im Niedersächsischen Justizvollzug. Oldenburg: Bibliotheks- und Informationssystem der Universität Oldenburg, 1996.

(Accepted 5 May 1998)

Getting research findings into practice
Barriers and bridges to evidence based clinical practice

Brian Haynes, Andrew Haines

Clinicians and healthcare planners who want to improve the quality and efficiency of healthcare services will find help in research evidence. This evidence is increasingly accessible through information services that combine high quality evidence with information technology. However, there are several barriers to the successful application of research evidence to health care. We discuss both the prospects for harnessing evidence to improve health care and the problems that readers—clinicians, planners, and patients—will need to overcome to enjoy the benefits of research (box).

The aim of evidence based health care is to provide the means by which current best evidence from research can be judiciously and conscientiously applied in the prevention, detection, and care of health disorders.[1] This aim is decidedly ambitious given how slowly important new treatments are disseminated into practice[2-4] and how resistant practitioners are to withdrawing established treatments from practice even once their utility has been disproved.[5]

The barriers to the dissemination and timely application of research findings in the making of decisions about health care are complex and have been little studied. They include many factors beyond the control of the practitioner and patient (such as being in the wrong place when illness occurs) as well as factors that might be modified to advantage (such as doing the wrong thing at the right time). Rather than attempting

Summary points

The aim of evidence based practice is to integrate current best evidence from research with clinical policy and practice

Practitioners have difficulty finding, assessing, interpreting, and applying current best evidence

New evidence based services (such as electronic databases, systematic reviews, and journals that summarise evidence) make accessing current best evidence feasible and easy in clinical settings

Progress is slow in creating evidence based clinical policy and in ensuring that evidence and policy are applied at the right time

This is the fourth in a series of eight articles analysing the gap between research and practice

Faculty of Health Sciences, McMaster University, 1200 Main St West, Hamilton, Ontario, Canada L8N 3Z5
Brian Haynes, *professor of clinical epidemiology and medicine*

Department of Primary Care and Population Sciences, Royal Free and University College London Schools of Medicine, London NW3 2PF
Andrew Haines, *professor of primary health care*

Correspondence to: Professor Haynes bhaynes@fhs. mcmaster.ca

Series editors: Andrew Haines and Anna Donald

BMJ 1998;317:273–6

Problems in implementing evidence based medicine and possible solutions

Problem	Solution
• The size and complexity of the research	Use services that abstract and synthesise information
• Difficulties in developing evidence based clinical policy	Produce guidelines for how to develop evidence based clinical guidelines
• Difficulties in applying evidence in practice because of the following factors:	
Poor access to best evidence and guidelines	Use information systems that integrate evidence and guidelines with patient care
Organisational barriers	Develop facilities and incentives to encourage effective care and better disease management systems
Ineffectual continuing education programmes	Improve effectiveness of educational and quality improvement programmes for practitioners
Low patient adherence to treatments	Develop more effective strategies to encourage patients to follow healthcare advice

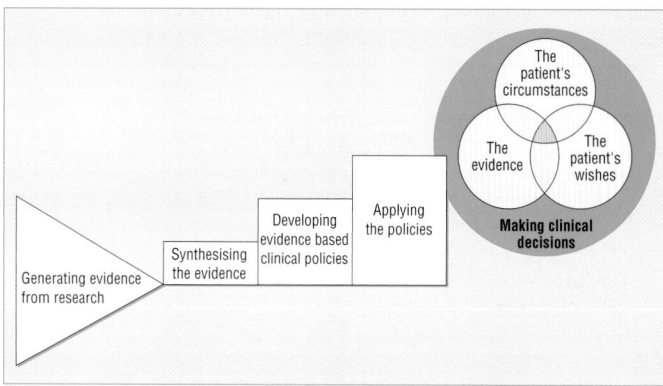

The path from the generation of evidence to the application of evidence

to dissect all these barriers, we present a simple model of the path (figure) along which evidence might travel to assist practitioners in making timely healthcare decisions. We will consider some barriers along this path and some bridges that are being constructed over the barriers.

Generating research evidence

The path begins with biomedical research: the shape of the wedge symbolises the process of testing innovations in health care and eliminating those that lack merit (figure). The broad edge of the wedge represents the initial testing of innovations, which usually occurs in laboratories; many new products and processes are discarded early in the testing process. Products or processes with merit then undergo field trials; these initial studies aim to assess toxicity and to estimate efficacy. Many innovations fail, but a few merit more definitive testing in large controlled trials with important clinical endpoints. It is only when studies are successful that serious efforts at dissemination and application are warranted. Increasingly, behavioural interventions, surgical procedures, and alternative approaches to the organisation and delivery of care are being subjected to similarly rigorous evaluation.

The biomedical and applied research enterprise represented by the wedge is vigorous, with an annual investment of over $55bn (£34.4bn) worldwide.[6] The amount of money spent on research provides hope

that healthcare services can be improved despite cutbacks in spending that are occurring in many countries. Unfortunately, many loose connections exist between research efforts and clinical practice, not the least of which is that preliminary studies far outnumber definitive ones, and all compete in the medical literature for the attention of readers.[7]

Steps from research to practice

The boxes to the right of the wedge (figure) represent the three steps that are needed to harness research evidence for healthcare practice. These steps include synthesising the evidence; developing clinical policy from the evidence; and applying the policy at the right place, in the right way, and at the right time. All three steps must be negotiated to form a valid connection between evidence and practice.

Synthesising the evidence

Most results from research appear first in peer reviewed journals, but the small number of clinically important studies are spread thinly through a vast number of publications; readers are bound to be overwhelmed. Models for critically appraising evidence have been developed and disseminated,[8] but applying these is time consuming. The newest bridges that can be used to overcome this barrier include abstracting services that critically appraise studies in which the results are ready to be applied to clinical settings; these appraisals are then summarised in a journal.[9 10] Many more of these new types of journals are being developed so that eventually most clinical specialties will have their own. More importantly, the Cochrane Collaboration has pledged to summarise all randomised controlled trials of healthcare interventions, and *The Cochrane Library* is now a robust resource.[11]

Along with these new services, advances in information technology can provide quick and often inexpensive access to high quality research evidence at the patient's bedside, in the clinician's office, or at the clinician's home.[8 12] Computerised decision support systems are maturing and allowing research findings to be taken one step further by fitting the evidence into patient specific reminders and aids to decision making embedded in clinical information systems.[13] These innovations are making the practice of evidence based health care much more feasible.

Creating evidence based clinical policies

To be both evidence based and clinically useful, clinical policy must balance the strengths and limitations of all relevant research evidence with the practical realities of the healthcare and clinical settings.[14] This is a problematic step because of limitations in both the evidence that is available and in policy making. Clinical practice guidelines developed by national groups may help individual practitioners but the expertise, will, resources, and effort required to ensure that they are scientifically sound as well as clinically helpful are in short supply, as witnessed by the conflicting guidelines issued by various professional bodies.[15] National healthcare policies are often moulded by a range of non-evidence based factors including historical, cultural, and ideological influences. Moreover, when national guidelines or healthcare policies encourage

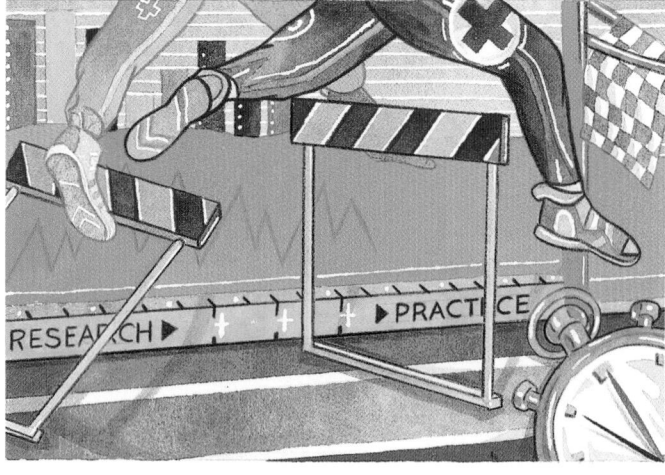

clinicians to perform procedures that are not evidence based, the unnecessary work acts as a barrier to the implementation of other well founded knowledge.

"Guidelines for guidelines" have been developed that will help if followed.[16] Evidence and guidelines must be understood by practitioners if they are to be applied well; understanding new material is a slow process that is not aided by traditional continuing education offerings.[17] Additionally, local and individual circumstances of clinical practice often affect the delivery of care, and national guidelines must be tailored to local circumstances by local practitioners; this tailoring of guidelines to local circumstances is a process that is only just beginning to occur.[18] Evidence can be used by individual practitioners to make policies, but few practitioners have the time and skill to derive policies from research evidence. The difficulties in developing sound policies are perhaps the greatest barriers to the implementation of research findings. Clinicians are in the best position to be able to balance research evidence with clinical circumstances, and must think and act as part of the team planning for change if progress is to be made.

Applying evidence based policy in practice

The next step in getting from research to practice is to apply evidence based policy at the right time, in the right place, and in the right way. Again, there are barriers at the local and individual levels. For example, for thrombolysis for acute myocardial infarction to be delivered within the brief time in which it is effective, the patient must recognise the symptoms, get to the hospital (avoiding a potentially delaying call to the family physician), and be seen right away by a health professional who recognises the problem and initiates treatment. For many people in many places this is still not happening.[19 20]

In some cases, particularly for surgery and other skilled procedures such as invasive diagnostic testing, a lack of training may constitute a barrier to implementing research findings. The complexity of guidelines may also thwart their application.[21] Organisational barriers to change must also be dealt with, for example, by ensuring that general practitioners have access to echocardiography to diagnose heart failure before starting treatment with angiotensin converting enzyme inhibitors.[22] Changes in the organisation of care (including in disease management), improvements in continuing education, interventions to improve quality among practitioners,[17] and improvements in computerised decision support systems,[13] are beginning to make inroads into the last steps that connect research evidence with practice. Unfortunately, these may all be undermined by limitations in the resources available for health services. Additionally, inappropriate economic measures may be used to evaluate healthcare programmes[23] though cost effective interventions may require considerable initial investment and have delayed benefits (this is especially true in the implementation of preventive procedures).

Making clinical decisions

Once the evidence has been delivered to the practitioner and the practitioner has recalled the evidence correctly and at the right place and time,

there are still steps to be taken. Firstly, the practitioner must define each patient's unique circumstances; this includes determining what is wrong with the patient and assessing how it is affecting the patient. For example, the cost effectiveness of lowering cholesterol concentrations with statins is highly dependent on the patient's own risk of adverse outcomes.[24] Secondly, the practitioner must then ask if the patient has any other problems that might influence the decision of which treatment is likely to be safe and effective. For example, carotid endarterectomy is highly effective for symptomatic carotid stenosis[25] but patients must be physically fit enough to have surgery. Evaluating the patient's clinical circumstances requires clinical expertise, without which no amount of research evidence will suffice.

Also, and increasingly, the patient's preferences, values, and rights are entering into the process of deciding on appropriate management. Thus, patients who are averse to immediate risk or cost may decline surgical procedures, such as endarterectomy, that offer longer term benefits even if they are physically fit to have surgery. Research evidence must be integrated with the patient's clinical circumstances and wishes to derive a meaningful decision about management, a process that no cookbook can describe. Indeed, everyone is still ignorant about the art of clinical practice. Although there is some evidence that exploring patients' experiences of illness may lead to improvements in their outcomes,[26] more research is needed into how to improve communication between clinicians and patients if we are to enhance progress in achieving evidence based health care. Additionally, there is a growing body of information available to patients that is both scientifically sound and intelligible, and many consumer and patient groups have made such material widely available.[27] Interactive media are being used (but not widely) to provide information to assist patients in making decisions about options for diagnosis and treatment.[28]

Finally, patients must follow the prescribed treatment plan; increasingly they are doing this independently because of the availability of effective treatments that allow ambulatory, self administered care, and also because of cutbacks in health services that necessitate more self care. We can help patients continue their care, but we are not so successful in helping them to follow our prescriptions closely, which dissipates much of the benefit of treatment.[29]

Conclusion

Successfully bridging the barriers between research evidence and clinical decision making will not ensure that patients receive optimal treatment; there are many other factors that might prevail, for example, the underfunding of health services and the maldistribution of resources. Nevertheless, incorporating current best evidence into clinical decision making promises to decrease the traditional delay between the generation of evidence and its application, and to increase the proportion of patients to whom current best treatment is offered. Quick access to accurate summaries of the best evidence is rapidly improving. The means for creating evidence based clinical policy and applying this policy judiciously and conscientiously are under development with help from health services research and information research.

1 Sackett DL, Rosenberg WMC, Gray JAM, Haynes RB. Evidence based medicine: what it is and what it isn't. *BMJ* 1996;312:71-2.
2 Mair F, Crowley T, Bundred P. Prevalence, aetiology and management of heart failure in general practice. *Br J Gen Pract* 1996;46:77-9.
3 Mashru M, Lant A. Interpractice audit of diagnosis and management of hypertension in primary care: educational intervention and review of medical records. *BMJ* 1997;314:942-6.
4 Sudlow M, Rodgers H, Kenny R, Thomson R. Population based study of use of anticoagulants among patients with atrial fibrillation in the community. *BMJ* 1997;314:1529-30.
5 Antman EM, Lau J, Kupelnick B, Mosteller F, Chalmers TC. A comparison of results of meta-analyses of randomized control trials and recommendations of experts. *JAMA* 1992;268:240-8.
6 Michaud C, Murray CJL. Resources for health research and development in 1992: a global overview. In: *Investing in health research and development: report of the ad hoc committee on health research relating to future intervention options.* Geneva: World Health Organisation, 1996:217.
7 Haynes RB. Loose connections between peer reviewed clinical journals and clinical practice. *Ann Intern Med* 1990;113:724-8.
8 Sackett DL, Richardson SR, Rosenberg W, Haynes RB. *Evidence-based medicine: how to practice and teach EBM.* London: Churchill Livingstone, 1997.
9 Haynes RB. The origins and aspirations of ACP Journal Club. *Ann Intern Med* 1991;114 (suppl 1):A18. (ACP Journal Club.)
10 Sackett DL, Haynes RB. On the need for evidence-based medicine. *Evidence-Based Med* 1995;1:5.
11 *The Cochrane Library* [database on disk and CD ROM]. Cochrane Collaboration. Oxford: Update Software; 1996-. Updated quarterly.
12 Hersh W. Evidence-based medicine and the internet. *ACP J Club* July-Aug 1996;125:A14-6.
13 Johnston ME, Langton KB, Haynes RB, Mathieu A. Effects of computer-based clinical decision support systems on clinician performance and patient outcome. A critical appraisal of research. *Ann Intern Med* 1994;120:135-42.
14 Gray JAM, Haynes RB, Sackett DL, Cook DJ, Guyatt GH. Transferring evidence from health care research into medical practice. 3. Developing evidence-based clinical policy. *Evidence-Based Med* 1997;2:36-8.
15 Krahn M, Naylor CD, Basinski AS, Detsky AS. Comparison of an aggressive (US) and a less aggressive (Canadian) policy for cholesterol screening and treatment. *Ann Intern Med* 1991;115:248-55.
16 Carter A. Background to the "guidelines for guidelines" series. *Can Med Assoc J* 1993;148:383.
17 Davis DA, Thomson MA, Oxman AD, Haynes RB. Changing physician performance: a systematic review of the effect of educational strategies. *JAMA* 1995;274:700-5.
18 Karuza J, Calkins E, Feather J, Hershey CD, Katz L, Majeroni B. Enhancing physician adoption of practice guidelines: dissemination of influenza vaccination guideline using a small-group consensus process. *Arch Intern Med* 1995;155:625-32.
19 Doorey AJ, Michelson EL, Topol EJ. Thrombolytic therapy of acute myocardial infarction. *JAMA* 1992;268:3108-14.
20 Ketley D, Woods KL. Impact of clinical trials on clinical practice: example of thrombolysis for acute myocardial infarction. *Lancet* 1993;342:891-4.
21 Grilli R, Lomas J. Evaluating the message: the relationship between compliance rate and the subject of a practice guideline. *Med Care* 1994;132:202-13.
22 Aszkenasy OM, Dawson D, Gill M, Haines A, Patterson DLH. Audit of direct access cardiac investigations: experience in an inner London health district. *J R Soc Med* 1994;87:588-90.
23 Sutton M. How to get the best health outcome for a given amount of money. *BMJ* 1997;315:47-9.
24 Pharoah PD, Hollingworth W. Cost effectiveness of lowering cholesterol concentration with statins in patients with and without pre-existing coronary heart disease: life table method applied to health authority population. *BMJ* 1996;312:1443-8.
25 European Carotid Surgery Trialists' Collaborative Group. MRC European carotid surgery trial: interim results for symptomatic patients with severe (70-99%) or with mild (0-29%) carotid stenosis. *Lancet* 1991;337:1235-43.
26 Stewart M. Studies of health outcomes and patient-centred communication. In: Stewart M, Brown JB, Weston WW, McWhinney IR, McWilliam CL, Freeman TR, eds. *Patient centred medicine.* Thousand Oaks, CA: Sage Publications, 1995:185-90.
27 Stocking B. Implementing the findings of effective care in pregnancy and childbirth. *Milbank Q* 1993;71:497-522.
28 Shepperd S, Coulter A, Farmer AU. Using interactive videos in general practice to inform patients about treatment choices. *Family Pract* 1995;12:443-7.
29 Haynes RB, McKibbon KA, Kanani R. Systematic review of randomised controlled trials of the effects on patient adherence and outcomes of interventions to assist patients to follow prescriptions for medications. *The Cochrane Library* [database on disk and CD ROM]. Cochrane Collaboration; 1997, Issue 2. Oxford: Update Software; 1997. Updated quarterly.

The articles in this series are adapted from *Getting Research Findings into Practice,* edited by Andrew Haines and Anna Donald and published by the BMJ Publishing Group

---

A memorable patient
Mountain power

Mark's cystic fibrosis was not diagnosed until he was 9 years old. When I first knew him, five years later, he already had advanced lung disease and was small for his age. Mark hated being small. He saw himself as "the little lad with the cough," a description he had once inadvertently overheard. Nevertheless, at this time, he had ambitions for his future and was extremely articulate about them, as indeed he was about everything.

After sitting his GCSEs at 16, Mark was longing for the sixth form. Sadly, he never made it. Instead he spent his last two and a half years mainly at home during which time he had to face all his aspirations, one by one, going out through the window as he became progressively more ill, chair bound, and eventually oxygen dependent. Despite this, Mark came to cope with a sort of growing inner peace.

There were many factors responsible for Mark's remarkable degree of acceptance. Among them were his innate personality and the support of his parents. But they were convinced, and I agree with them, that an experience he had in his last term at school made a profoundly important contribution. This was a weekend spent with a group of his school mates at an organised retreat. A topic for discussion with an essay to write were a part of it. The topic, ironically, was "What are my reasons for wanting to go on living."

I will never forget Mark's first outpatient attendance after that weekend. He looked just as wan and ill as ever but there was a radiance about him I had never seen before. I asked him what had happened. He told me that he had had this wonderful weekend which had "restored his confidence in himself." The only incident of the weekend he recounted at the time was of an outing on the last afternoon to climb a mountain.

Now, there was no way that Mark could climb a mountain; that was crystal clear to everyone, but it seemed that there was no way that these young people would allow him not to climb the mountain. So they carried him up. One by one, one after another, they put him on their shoulders and carried him up until, on reaching the top, Mark was higher than anyone else.

This taught Mark a lot of things. In particular, in relating to people, his age and illness did not matter. Also, that if he could accept help, not easy at 16, it paid dividends. In fact, for the remainder of his life that mountain experience became symbolic for us both in facing and overcoming setbacks.

But that was not all. It was only after Mark's death that his parents found the notebook from that weekend. In it was his essay on why he wanted to go on living. In this he described how he wanted to become an independent person, not just "the little lad with the cough." At the back of the notebook every child who was there had written a personal tribute to Mark about his courage and his personality. These sincere and undoubtedly unexpected tributes must have done much to restore Mark's battered self image and, as he put it, his "confidence in himself."

Mark, so articulate and so anxious to talk, gave me an invaluable insight into what it meant for a bright, achieving youngster to face a progressively disabling illness and untimely death. His was the voice which spoke for all children, similarly placed, who were unable or reluctant to talk about themselves.

Olive McKendrick, *retired paediatrician, Liverpool*

We welcome articles up to 600 words on topics such as *A memorable patient, A paper that changed my practice, My most unfortunate mistake,* or any other piece conveying instruction, pathos, or humour. If possible the article should be supplied on a disk. Permission is needed from the patient or a relative if an identifiable patient is referred to. We also welcome contributions for "Endpieces," consisting of quotations of up to 80 words (but most are considerably shorter) from any source, ancient or modern, which have appealed to the reader.

1   Department of Health. *Changing childbirth: the report of the Expert Maternity Group.* London: HMSO, 1993.
2   Pinkerton JV, Finnerty LL. Resolving the clinical and ethical dilemma involved in fetal-maternal conflicts. *Am J Obstet Gynecol* 1996;175:289-95.
3   Bolaji II, Meehan FP. Post caesarean delivery. *Eur J Gynaecol Obstet Reprod Biol* 1993;51:181-92.
4   Meehan FP, Rafla NM, Bolaji II. Delivery following previous caesarean section. In: Studd J, ed. *Progress in obstetrics and gynaecology.* Vol 10. London: Churchill Livingstone, 1993:213-28.
5   Savage W, Francome C. British caesarean section rates: have we reached a plateau? *Br J Obstet Gynaecol* 1993;100:493-6.
6   Sultan AH, Kamm MA, Hudson CN, Thomas JM, Bartram CI. Anal sphincter disruption during vaginal delivery. *N Engl J Med* 1993;329:1905-11.
7   Sultan AH, Kamm MA, Hudson CN, Bartram CI. Third degree obstetric anal sphincter tears: risk factors and outcome of primary repair. *BMJ* 1994;308:887-91.
8   Al-Mufti R, McCarthy A, Fisk NM. Obstetricians' personal choice and mode of delivery. *Lancet* 1996;347:544.
9   Dolan B, Parker C; Bowley S; Whitfield A; Bastian H, Conroy C. Caesarean section: a treatment for mental disorder? *BMJ* 1997;314:1183-7.
10 Snooks SJ, Swash M, Mathers SE, Henry MM. Effect of vaginal delivery on the pelvic floor: a 5-year follow up. *Br J Surg* 1990;77:1358-60.
11 Weinstein D, Benshushan A, Tanos V, Zilberstein R, Rojansky N. Predictive score for vaginal birth after caesarean section. *Am J Obstet Gynecol* 1996;174:192-8.
12 Sultan AH, Stanton SL. Preserving the pelvic floor and perineum during childbirth—elective caesarean section? *Br J Obstet Gynaecol* 1996;103:731-4.
13 Hemminki E, Merilainen J. Long-term effects of caesarean section: ectopic pregnancies and placental problems. *Am J Obstet Gynaecol* 1996;174:1569-74.
14 NHS Executive. *Consent to treatment; summary of legal rulings.* Wetherby: Department of Health, 1997. (Executive letter EL(97)32.)
15 What is the right number of caesarean sections? [editorial]. *Lancet* 1997;349:815.

Getting research findings into practice

Closing the gap between research and practice: an overview of systematic reviews of interventions to promote the implementation of research findings

Lisa A Bero, Roberto Grilli, Jeremy M Grimshaw, Emma Harvey, Andrew D Oxman, Mary Ann Thomson on behalf of the Cochrane Effective Practice and Organisation of Care Review Group

Despite the considerable amount of money spent on clinical research relatively little attention has been paid to ensuring that the findings of research are implemented in routine clinical practice.[1] There are many different types of intervention that can be used to promote behavioural change among healthcare professionals and the implementation of research findings. Disentangling the effects of intervention from the influence of contextual factors is difficult when interpreting the results of individual trials of behavioural change.[2] Nevertheless, systematic reviews of rigorous studies provide the best evidence of the effectiveness of different strategies for promoting behavioural change.[3 4] In this paper we examine systematic reviews of different strategies for the dissemination and implementation of research findings to identify evidence of the effectiveness of different strategies and to assess the quality of the systematic reviews.

Identification and inclusion of systematic reviews

We searched Medline records dating from 1966 to June 1995 using a strategy developed in collaboration with the NHS Centre for Reviews and Dissemination. The search identified 1139 references. No reviews from the Cochrane Effective Practice and Organisation of Care Review Group[4] had been published during this time. In addition, we searched the *Database of Abstracts of Research Effectiveness* (DARE) (www.york.ac.uk/inst/crd) but did not identify any other review meeting the inclusion criteria.

We searched for any review of interventions to improve professional performance that reported explicit selection criteria and in which the main outcomes considered were changes in performance or outcome. Reviews that did not report explicit selection

Summary points

Systematic reviews of rigorous studies provide the best evidence on the effectiveness of different strategies to promote the implementation of research findings

Passive dissemination of information is generally ineffective

It seems necessary to use specific strategies to encourage implementation of research based recommendations and to ensure changes in practice

Further research on the relative effectiveness and efficiency of different strategies is required

criteria, systematic reviews focusing on the methodological quality of published studies, published bibliographies, bibliographic databases, and registers of projects on dissemination activities were excluded from our review. If systematic reviews had been updated we considered only the most recently published review. For example, the *Effective Health Care* bulletin on implementing clinical guidelines superseded the earlier review by Grimshaw and Russell.[5 6]

Two reviewers independently assessed the quality of the reviews and extracted data on the focus, inclusion criteria, main results, and conclusions of each review. A previously validated checklist (including nine criteria scored as done, partially done, or not done) was used to assess quality.[7 8] Reviews also gave a summary score (out of seven) based on the scientific quality of the review. Major disagreements between reviewers were resolved by discussion and consensus.

This is the seventh in a series of eight articles analysing the gap between research and practice

Institute for Health Policy Studies, University of California at San Francisco, 1388 Sutter Street, 11th floor, San Francisco, CA 94109, USA
Lisa A Bero, *associate professor*
Unit of Clinical Policy Analysis, Laboratory of Clinical Epidemiology, Istituto di Ricerche Farmacologiche Mario Negri, Via Eritrea 62, 20157 Milan, Italy
Roberto Grilli, *head*

continued over

BMJ 1998;317:465–8

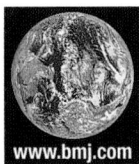

www.bmj.com

Additional data can be found on our website

Health Services
Research Unit,
Department of
Public Health,
Aberdeen
AB25 2ZD
Jeremy M
Grimshaw,
programme director
Mary Ann
Thomson,
senior research fellow

Department of
Health Sciences
and Clinical
Evaluation,
University of York,
York YO1 5DD
Emma Harvey,
research fellow

Health Services
Research Unit,
National Institute of
Public Health, PO
Box 4404 Torshov,
N-0462 Oslo,
Norway
Andrew D Oxman,
director

Correspondence to:
Dr Grimshaw
j.m.grimshaw@
abdn.ac.uk

Series editors:
Andrew Haines and
Anna Donald

Results and assessment of systematic reviews

We identified 18 reviews that met the inclusion criteria. They were categorised as focusing on broad strategies (such as the dissemination and implementation of guidelines[5 6 9-11]), continuing medical education,[12 13] particular strategies (such as audit and feedback,[14 15] computerised decision support systems,[16 17] or multi-faceted interventions[18]), particular target groups (for example, nurses[19] or primary healthcare professionals[20]), and particular problem areas or types of behaviour (for example, diagnostic testing,[15] prescribing,[21] or aspects of preventive care[15 22-25]). Most primary studies were included in more than one review, and some reviewers published more than one review. No systematic reviews published before 1988 were identified. None of the reviews explicitly addressed the cost effectiveness of different strategies for effecting changes in behaviour.

There was a lack of a common approach adopted between the reviews in how interventions and potentially confounding factors were categorised. The inclusion criteria and methods used in these reviews varied considerably. Interventions were frequently classed differently in the different systematic reviews.

Common methodological problems included the failure to adequately report criteria for selecting studies included in the review, the failure to avoid bias in the selection of studies, the failure to adequately report criteria used to assess validity, and the failure to apply criteria to assess the validity of the selected studies. Overall, 42% (68/162) of criteria were reported as having been done, 49% (80/162) as having been partially done, and 9% (14/162) as not having been done. The mean summary score was 4.13 (range 2 to 6, median 3.75, mode 3).

Encouragingly, reviews published more recently seemed to be of better quality. For studies published between 1988 and 1991 (n=6) only 20% (11/54) of criteria were scored as having been done (mean summary score 3.0); for reviews published after 1991 (n=12) 52% (56/108) of criteria were scored as having been done (mean summary score 4.7).

Five reviews attempted formal meta-analyses of the results of the studies identified.[12 17 19 23 25] The appropriateness of meta-analysis in three of these reviews is

uncertain,[12 17 19] and the reviews should be considered exploratory at best, given the broad focus and heterogeneity of the studies included in the reviews with respect to the types of interventions, targeted behaviours, contextual factors, and other research factors.[2]

A number of consistent themes were identified by the systematic reviews (box). (Further details about the systematic reviews are available on the *BMJ*'s website.) Most of the reviews identified modest improvements in performance after interventions. However, the passive dissemination of information was generally ineffective in altering practices no matter how important the issue or how valid the assessment methods.[5 9 11 13 21 26] The use of computerised decision support systems has led to improvements in the performance of doctors in terms of decisions on drug dosage, the provision of preventive care, and the general clinical management of patients, but not in diagnosis.[16] Educational outreach visits have resulted in improvements in prescribing decisions in North America.[5 13] Patient mediated interventions also seem to improve the provision of preventive care in North America (where baseline performance is often very low).[13] Multifaceted interventions (that is, a combination of methods that includes two or more interventions such as participation in audit and a local consensus process) seem to be more effective than single interventions.[13 18] There is insufficient evidence to assess the effectiveness of some interventions—for example the identification and recruitment of local opinion leaders (practitioners nominated by their colleagues as influential).[5]

Few reviews attempted explicitly to link their findings to theories of behavioural change. The difficulties associated with linking findings and theories are illustrated in the review by Davis et al, who found that the results of their overview supported several different theories of behavioural change.[13]

Availability and quality of primary studies

This overview also allows the opportunity to estimate the availability and quality of primary research in the areas of dissemination and implementation. Identification of published studies on behavioural change is difficult because they are poorly indexed and scattered across generalist and specialist journals. Nevertheless, two reviews provided an indication of the extent of research in this area. Oxman et al identified 102 randomised or quasirandomised controlled trials involving 160 comparisons of interventions to improve professional practice.[11] The *Effective Health Care* bulletin on implementing clinical guidelines identified 91 rigorous studies (including 63 randomised or quasirandomised controlled trials and 28 controlled before and after studies or time series analyses).[5] Even though the studies included in these two reviews fulfilled the minimum inclusion criteria, some are methodologically flawed and have potentially major threats to their validity. Many studies randomised health professionals or groups of professionals (cluster randomisation) but analysed the results by patient, thus resulting in a possible overestimation of the significance of the observed effects (unit of analysis error).[27] Given the small to moderate size of the observed effects this could lead to false conclusions about the significance of the effectiveness of interventions in

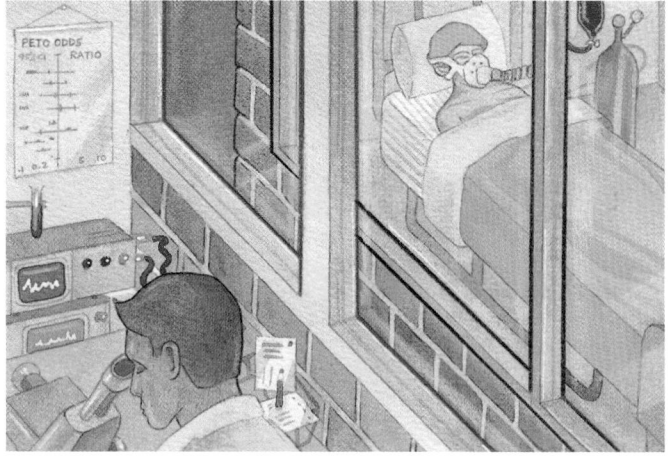

IAN BARRACLOUGH

Interventions to promote behavioural change among health professionals

Consistently effective interventions
- Educational outreach visits (for prescribing in North America)
- Reminders (manual or computerised)
- Multifaceted interventions (a combination that includes two or more of the following: audit and feedback, reminders, local consensus processes, or marketing)
- Interactive educational meetings (participation of healthcare providers in workshops that include discussion or practice)

Interventions of variable effectiveness
- Audit and feedback (or any summary of clinical performance)
- The use of local opinion leaders (practitioners identified by their colleagues as influential)
- Local consensus processes (inclusion of participating practitioners in discussions to ensure that they agree that the chosen clinical problem is important and the approach to managing the problem is appropriate)
- Patient mediated interventions (any intervention aimed at changing the performance of healthcare providers for which specific information was sought from or given to patients)

Interventions that have little or no effect
- Educational materials (distribution of recommendations for clinical care, including clinical practice guidelines, audiovisual materials, and electronic publications)
- Didactic educational meetings (such as lectures)

both meta-analyses and qualitative analyses. Few studies attempted to undertake any form of economic analysis.

Given the importance of implementing the results of sound research and the problems of generalisability across different healthcare settings, there are relatively few studies of individual interventions to effect behavioural change. The review by Oxman et al identified studies involving 12 comparisons of educational materials, 17 of conferences, four of outreach visits, six of local opinion leaders, 10 of patient mediated interventions, 33 of audit and feedback, 53 of reminders, two of marketing, eight of local consensus processes, and 15 of multifaceted interventions.[11] Few studies compared the relative effectiveness of different strategies; only 22 out of 91 studies reviewed in the *Effective Health Care* bulletin allowed comparisons of different strategies.[5] A further limitation of the evidence about different types of interventions is that the research is often conducted by limited numbers of researchers in specific settings. The generalisability of these findings to other settings is uncertain, especially because of the marked differences in undergraduate and postgraduate education, the organisation of healthcare systems, potential systemic incentives and barriers to change, and societal values and cultures. Most of the studies reviewed were conducted in North America; only 14 of the 91 studies reviewed in the *Effective Health Care* bulletin had been conducted in Europe.[5]

The way forward

This overview suggests that there is an increasing amount of primary and secondary research in the areas of dissemination and implementation. It is striking how little is known about the effectiveness and cost effectiveness of interventions that aim to change the practice or delivery of health care. The reviews that we examined suggest that the passive dissemination of information (for example, publication of consensus conferences in professional journals or the mailing of educational materials) is generally ineffective and, at best, results only in small changes in practice. However, these passive approaches probably represent the most common approaches adopted by researchers, professional bodies, and healthcare organisations. The use of specific strategies to implement research based recommendations seems to be necessary to ensure that practices change, and studies suggest that more intensive efforts to alter practice are generally more successful.

At a local level greater attention needs to be given to actively coordinating dissemination and implementation to ensure that research findings are implemented. The choice of intervention should be guided by the evidence on the effectiveness of dissemination and implementation strategies, the characteristics of the message,[10] the recognition of external barriers to change,[13] and the preparedness of the clinicians to change.[28] Local policymakers with responsibility for professional education or quality assurance need to be aware of the results of implementation research, develop expertise in the principles of the management of change, and accept the need for local experimentation.

Given the paucity of evidence it is vital that dissemination and implementation activities should be rigorously evaluated whenever possible. Studies evaluating a single intervention provide little new information about the relative effectiveness and cost effectiveness of different interventions in different settings. Greater emphasis should be given to conducting studies that evaluate two or more interventions in a specific setting or help clarify the circumstances that are likely to modify the effectiveness of an intervention. Economic evaluations should be considered an integral component of research. Researchers should have greater awareness of the issues related to cluster randomisation, and should ensure that studies have adequate power and that they are analysed using appropriate methods.[29]

The NHS research and development programme on evaluating methods to promote the implementation of research and development is an important initiative that will contribute to our knowledge of the dissemination of information and the implementation of research findings.[30] However, these research issues cut across national and cultural differences in the practice and financing of health care. Moreover, the scope of these issues is such that no one country's health services research programme can examine them in a comprehensive way. This suggests that there are potential benefits of international collaboration and cooperation in research, as long as appropriate attention is paid to cultural factors that might influence the implementation process such as the beliefs and perceptions of the public, patients, healthcare professionals, and policymakers.

123

The results of primary research should be systematically reviewed to identify promising implementation techniques and areas where more research is required.[3] Undertaking reviews in this area is difficult because of the complexity inherent in the interventions, the variability in the methods used, and the difficulty of generalising study findings across healthcare settings. The Cochrane Effective Practices and Organisation of Care Review Group is helping to meet the need for systematic reviews of current best evidence on the effects of continuing medical education, quality assurance, and other interventions that affect professional practice. A growing number of these reviews are being published and updated in the *Cochrane Database of Systematic Reviews*.[4 31]

This paper is based on a briefing paper prepared by the authors for the Advisory Group on the NHS research and development programme on evaluating methods to promote the implementation of research and development. We thank Nick Freemantle for his contribution to this paper.

Funding: This work was partly funded by the European Community funded Eur-Assess project. The Cochrane Effective Practice and Organisation of Care Review Group is funded by the Chief Scientist Office of the Scottish Office Home and Health Department; the NHS Welsh Office of Research and Development; the Northern Ireland Department of Health and Social Services; the research and development offices of the Anglia and Oxford, North Thames, North West, South and West, South Thames, Trent, and West Midlands regions; and by the Norwegian Research Council and Ministry of Health and Social Affairs in Norway. The Health Services Research Unit is funded by the Chief Scientist Office of the Scottish Office Home and Health Department. The views expressed are those of the authors and not necessarily the funding bodies.

Conflict of interest: None.

The articles in this series are adapted from *Getting Research Findings into Practice*, edited by Andrew Haines and Anna Donald and published by BMJ Books.

1 Eddy DM. Clinical policies and the quality of clinical practice. *N Engl J Med* 1982;307:343-7.
2 Grimshaw JM, Freemantle N, Langhorne P, Song F. *Complexity and systematic reviews: report to the US Congress Office of Technology Assessment.* Washington, DC: Office of Technology Assessment, 1995.
3 Mulrow CD. Rationale for systematic reviews. *BMJ* 1994;309:597-9.
4 Bero L, Grilli R, Grimshaw JM, Harvey E, Oxman AD, eds. Effective professional practice and organisation of care module, Cochrane Database of Systematic Reviews. *The Cochrane Library.* The Cochrane Collaboration; Issue 4. Oxford: Update Software; 1997.
5 Implementing clinical guidelines: can guidelines be used to improve clinical practice? *Effective Health Care* 1994; No 8.
6 Grimshaw JM, Russell IT. Effect of clinical guidelines on medical practice: a systematic review of rigorous evaluations. *Lancet* 1993;342:1317-22.
7 Oxman AD, Guyatt GH. The science of reviewing research. *Ann N Y Acad Sci* 1993;703:123-31.
8 Oxman AD. Checklists for review articles. *BMJ* 1994;309:648-51.
9 Lomas J. Words without action? The production, dissemination, and impact of consensus recommendations. *Annu Rev Public Health* 1991;12:41-65.
10 Grilli R, Lomas J. Evaluating the message: the relationship between compliance rate and the subject of a practice guideline. *Med Care* 1994;32:202-13.
11 Oxman AD, Thomson MA, Davis DA, Haynes RB. No magic bullets: a systematic review of 102 trials of interventions to help health care professionals deliver services more effectively or efficiently. *Can Med Assoc J* 1995;153:1423-31.
12 Beaudry JS. The effectiveness of continuing medical education: a quantitative synthesis. *J Continuing Education Health Professions* 1989;9:285-307.
13 Davis DA, Thomson MA, Oxman AD, Haynes RB. Changing physician performance: a systematic review of the effect of continuing medical education strategies. *JAMA* 1995;274:700-5.
14 Mugford M, Banfield P, O'Hanlon M. Effects of feedback of information on clinical practice: a review. *BMJ* 1991;303:398-402.
15 Buntinx F, Winkens R, Grol R, Knottnerus JA. Influencing diagnostic and preventive performance in ambulatory care by feedback and reminders: a review. *Fam Pract* 1993;10:219-28.
16 Johnston ME, Langton KB, Haynes RB, Mathieu A. Effects of computer-based clinical decision support systems on clinician performance and patient outcome: a critical appraisal of research. *Ann Intern Med* 1994;120:135-42.
17 Austin SM, Balas EA, Mitchell JA, Ewigman BG. Effect of physician reminders on preventive care: meta-analysis of randomized clinical trials. *Proceedings—the Annual Symposium on Computer Applications in Medical Care* 1994;121-4.
18 Wensing M, Grol R. Single and combined strategies for implementing changes in primary care: a literature review. *Int J Quality Health Care* 1994;6:115-32.
19 Waddell DL. The effects of continuing education on nursing practice: a meta-analysis. *J Continuing Education Nurs* 1991;22:113-8.
20 Yano EM, Fink A, Hirsch SH, Robbins AS, Rubenstein LV. Helping practices reach primary care goals: lessons from the literature. *Arch Intern Med* 1995;155:1146-56.
21 Soumerai SB, McLaughlin TJ, Avorn J. Improving drug prescribing in primary care: a critical analysis of the experimental literature. *Milbank Q* 1989;67:268-317.
22 Lomas J, Haynes RB. A taxonomy and critical review of tested strategies for the application of clinical practice recommendations: from "official" to "individual" clinical policy. *Am J Prev Med* 1987;4:77-94.
23 Gyorkos TW, Tannenbaum TN, Abrahamowicz M, Bédard L, Carsley J, Franco ED, et al. Evaluation of the effectiveness of immunization delivery methods. *Can J Public Health* 1994;85(suppl 1):14-30S.
24 Mandleblatt J, Kanetsky PA. Effectiveness of interventions to enhance physician screening for breast cancer. *J Fam Pract* 1995;40:162-71.
25 Silagy C, Lancaster T, Gray S, Fowler G. The effectiveness of training health professionals to provide smoking cessation interventions: systematic review of randomised controlled trials. *Qual Health Care* 1995;3:193-8.
26 Lomas J, Anderson GM, Domnick-Pierre K, Vayda E, Enkin MW, Hannah WJ. Do practice guidelines guide practice? The effect of a consensus statement on the practice of physicians. *N Engl J Med* 1989;321:1306-11.
27 Whiting-O'Keefe QE, Henke C, Simborg DW. Choosing the correct unit of analysis in medical care experiments. *Med Care* 1984;22:1101-14.
28 Grol R. Implementing guidelines in general practice care. *Qual Health Care* 1992;1:184-91.
29 Donner A, Birkett N, Buck C. Randomisation by cluster: sample size requirements and analysis. *Am J Epidemiol* 1981;114:906-14.
30 NHS Research and Development Programme. *Methods to promote the implementation of research findings in the NHS: priorities for evaluation.* Leeds: Department of Health, 1995.
31 Freemantle N, Grilli R, Grimshaw JM, Oxman A. Implementing the findings of medical research: the Cochrane Collaboration on effective professional practice. *Qual Health Care* 1995;4:45-7.

Statistics Notes

Time to event (survival) data

Douglas G Altman, J Martin Bland

Correspondence to: Mr Altman

continued over

BMJ 1998;317:468–9

In many medical studies an outcome of interest is the time to an event. Such events may be adverse, such as death or recurrence of a tumour; positive, such as conception or discharge from hospital; or neutral, such as cessation of breast feeding. It is conventional to talk about survival data and survival analysis, regardless of the nature of the event. Similar data also arise when measuring the time to complete a task, such as walking 50 metres.

The distinguishing feature of survival data is that at the end of the follow up period the event will probably not have occurred for all patients. For these patients the survival time is said to be censored, indicating that the observation period was cut off before the event occurred. We do not know when (or, indeed, whether) the patient will experience the event, only that he or she has not done so by the end of the observation period.

24 Anderson TJ, Rivest J, Stell R, Steiger MJ, Cohen H, Thompson PD, et al. Botulinum toxin treatment of spasmodic torticollis. *J R Soc Med* 1992;85:524-9.

25 Lepore V, Defazio G, Acquistapance P, Helpignano C, Powes L, Lambert P, et al. Botulinum A toxin for the so-called apraxia of lid opening. *Mov Disord* 1995;10:525-6.

26 Brin MF, Blitzer A, Steward C. Laryngeal dystonia (spasmodic dysphonia): observations of 901 patients and treatment with botulinum toxin. In: Fahn S, Marsden CD, DeLong MR, eds. *Advances in neurology. Dystonia*. Philadelphia: Lippincott-Raven, 1998:237-52.

27 Tsui JKC, Bhatt M, Calne S, Calne DB. Botulinum toxin in the treatment of writer's cramp: a double-blind study. *Neurology* 1993;43:183-5.

28 Jitpimolmard S, Tiamkao S, Laopaiboon M. Long term results of botulinum toxin type A (Dysport) in the treatment of hemifacial spasm: a report of 175 cases. *J Neurol Neurosurg Psychiatry* 1998;64:751-7.

29 Trosch RM, Pullman SL. Botulinum toxin A injections for the treatment of hand tremors. *Mov Disord* 1994;9:601-9.

30 Simpson DM. Clinical trials of botulinum toxin in the treatment of spasticity. *Muscle Nerve* 1997;20(suppl 6):S169-75.

31 Boyd R, Graham HK. Botulinum toxin A in the management of children with cerebral palsy: indications and outcome. *Eur J Neurol* 1997:4(suppl 2):S15-22.

32 Sheean GL. The treatment of spasticity with botulinum toxin. In: Sheean GL, Barnes MP, eds. *Spasticity rehabilitation*. London: Churchill Communications, 1998:109-26.

33 Maria G, Cassetta E, Gui D, Brisinda G, Bentivoglio AR, Albanese A. A comparison of botulinum toxin and saline for the treatment of chronic anal fissure. *N Engl J Med* 1998;338:217-20.

34 Cuillier C, Ducrotte P, Zerbib F, Metman EH, de Looze D, Guillemot F, et al. Achalasia: outcome of patients treated with intrasphincteric injection of botulinum toxin. *Gut* 1997;41:87-92.

35 Shelley WB, Talanin NY, Shelley ED. Botulinum toxin therapy for palmar hyperhidrosis. *J Am Acad Dermatol* 1998;38:227-9.

36 Naumann M, Zellner M, Toyka KV, Reiners K. Treatment of gustatory sweating with botulinum toxin. *Ann Neurol* 1997;42:973-5.

37 Bhatia KP, Münchau A, Brown P. Botulinum toxin is a useful treatment in extensive drooling of saliva. *J Neurol Neurosurg Psychiatry* 1999;67:697.

(Accepted 16 August 1999)

Evidence based case report

Asymptomatic haematuria ... in the doctor

Chris Del Mar

The patient was waiting in the consulting room; everything was nearly ready. The occasion was the examination in general practice for fifth year medical students. We run an objective structured clinical examination. For this part, the student had to measure the patient's blood pressure (the "patient" was actually someone recruited from our general practice), test his urine using a dipstick, and report to the examiner within the five minutes between bells. Just one thing was missing—the midstream sample of normal urine for testing. Because I did not want to disturb the volunteer patient, I collected it from myself. I measured the patient's blood pressure again (this had to be done after every 10th student)—it was stable. And I tested the urine to check it was normal—it was not.

For the next two hours, students either told me (or, in the case of those less skilled at this technique, did not tell me) that there was a trace of blood in the urine. This was not a problem as far as the examination was concerned because the marking was not affected by the test result. But it was a problem for me. What should I do? I tested my urine again a week later, and when I found it was still positive I sent a specimen to the laboratory. The report stated that urine culture was negative but confirmed the presence of normal red cells (30/ml).

Conventional medical teaching had taught me that bleeding must come from somewhere. The model that sprang to mind first is summarised in the table. I then checked with a textbook of surgery.[1] I had forgotten tuberculosis and schistosomiasis as causes of haematuria. A textbook of medicine[2] suggested further assessments, including checking my blood relatives for urine abnormality and carrying out haemoglobin electrophoresis and 24 hour urinary estimations of urate and calcium excretion. If all these investigations were negative, intravenous urography, cystoscopy, and renal computed tomography were proposed, with indefinite regular follow up thereafter. The essential feature of this model is that identifying the lesion anatomically or physiologically is the key to managing the problem. Early diagnosis of some of the serious causes of

haematuria such as transitional cell carcinoma might affect the outcome favourably by enabling treatment to be given. With other causes such as minimal change glomerulonephritis, early diagnosis is unlikely to affect mortality or morbidity.

I consulted my general practice colleague. His approach was similar. He ensured that I had checked my urine microscopy and culture to establish whether the blood was haemolysed or not, and he measured my blood pressure. He wondered whether my bicycle riding might be the cause, and suggested I recheck the urine after a month or two. If test results were still positive, it looked as if the cascade of likely events would include ultrasonography, urine samples for malignant cells, and then probably referral to a urologist for consideration of cystoscopy and intravenous urography.

"We probably won't find any cause for it," he said. I think this was to reassure me. I had time to think about adopting an evidence based approach.

Formulating the question

The most difficult part of adopting evidence in practice is formulating the question. This involves quite a different way in thinking—away from "patho-anatomical-physiological" questions towards empirical ones. What is the chance of having a serious condition with asymptomatic haematuria? What sort of study did I want? Ideally, it would be huge study of general

Centre for General Practice, University of Queensland, The University General Practice, Inala, Queensland 4077, Australia
Chris Del Mar *professor*
c.delmar@mailbox.uq.edu.au

BMJ 2000;320:165–6

Causes and management of haematuria

Site of bleeding	Disease	Management
Generalised	Bleeding diathesis	Check bleeding and coagulation profiles; treat accordingly
Lower renal tract	Prostate hypertrophy or cancer; urethral inflammation; bladder lesion or cancer	Cystoscopy; treat accordingly
Ureteric lesions	Transitional cell carcinoma; ureteric calculi	Ultrasonography or intravenous urography; treat accordingly
Renal lesions	Cancer; calculi; vascular abnormalities; reflux nephropathy; glomerular lesions	Check blood pressure; ultrasonography or intravenous urography; treat accordingly

practice academics in their 40s who had unexpectedly found haematuria during their academic duties. And the outcome would be a cohort study with a long follow up to see what illness occurred.

Searching for evidence

The standard textbooks on my shelf were no help in providing the evidence, so I consulted *The Cochrane Library* (on CD Rom). This would have been the most convenient source of data and is strong on evidence for different treatments, but unfortunately it does not yet include routinely collected data on the course of diseases and conditions. Since *The Cochrane Library* did not help, I decided to search Medline. My search strategy was simple,[3] and probably sensitive at the expense of being less specific: the term used was "(incidence or explode (mortality or (follow-up studies) or mortality or prognosis: or predict: or course)) and (hematuria or haematuria)."

Inspection of titles helped me discard immediately about half the 230 hits, but reading through the printout of abstracts of the remainder took an evening. There were no systematic reviews—the best form of evidence.[4] Two articles were clearly useful because they described large studies with long term follow up of people with negative and positive dipstick test results. I obtained the full versions of the papers from the library.

The evidence

In a British study, 2.5% of more than 10 000 men screened for asymptomatic haematuria by dipstick testing had positive results, of whom 60% were investigated further by their general practitioners.[5] Three had a serious condition that was amenable to cure—two had bladder cancer and one had reflux nephropathy. This study seemed to be fairly close to my ideal. It gave a prognosis of the outcome someone like me (my situation being similar to screening) would expect. It suggested that I was unlikely to have a serious condition that was amenable to cure. Of course, even this may be an overestimate of the benefits of screening. Perhaps those three people would have developed symptoms such as frank haematuria or dysuria sufficiently early to negate the beneficial effect of screening on their prognosis.

Another study was done in California.[6] Over 20 000 middle aged people were screened by dipstick for haematuria. An unexpected positive result was found in nearly 3%, 99% of whom were followed up. Over the next three years, three patients developed urological cancers (two prostatic and one bladder). This study is more relevant because it looked at the outcome of people whose dipstick test was not positive; their probability of developing urological cancer was no less than that of people whose dipstick test was positive. According to this study, the likelihood of my developing urological cancer was 0.5%, whether I had haematuria or not.

Were the studies of good enough quality? As they were studies of patients selected for screening, they were probably the best match with my situation that I could hope for. The second study, particularly, seemed to address a variety of potential selection biases. In the absence of a formal meta-analysis, this seemed to be a sufficiently serious "dip" into the published reports to answer my clinical question.

Another study on young men in the air force shed a little light on factors associated with microscopic haematuria. Neither exercise, recent sexual intercourse, nor flying were associated with microscopic haematuria, although recall of a history of urethritis was.[7] My bicycling was probably unrelated.

The clinical decision

What should I do now? I decided that the chance of having an adverse outcome was not sufficiently high for me to bother with further investigations. I would adopt a management policy of "expectant observation." I have watched for frank haematuria or any other new signs, and I check my urine every three months (the haematuria has remained, but there has been no increase in the concentration of red cells over the past year).

I have applied my own values to the clinical decision. If, in similar circumstances, a patient of mine elected to proceed with further investigations, I would comply. This does not address matters of gatekeeping (resource allocation), which probably should be dealt with away from the consultation.

Discussion

How has an evidence based approach helped? The main difference was the change in clinical thinking that allowed me to break away from the patho-anatomical-physiological approach and adopt an empirical one. These steps are not easy. Searching the published reports is still awkward and time consuming. Some answers are difficult to find. How long, for example, should we carry on looking before concluding that there seems to be no published work to guide us? We also need a forum of peers and those skilled at evidence based medicine in which test out our ideas so that we can reassure ourselves that we are not completely off course. If health authorities are serious about promoting evidence based medicine in clinical practice, they may have to consider providing a service (perhaps like pathology, radiology, or referred specialist opinions) to help clinicians to take these steps.

Paul Glasziou constructively read earlier drafts and checked, with Geoff Hirst, that I was not completely off course; my thanks to both.

Funding: None.

Competing interests: None declared.

1 Tipcraft RC. Urinary symptoms. Investigation of the urinary tract. Anuria. In: Mann CV, Russell RCG, William NS, eds. *Bailey and Love's short practice of surgery*. London: Chapman and Hall Medical, 1995:904-14.
2 Denker BM, Brenner BM. Cardinal management of renal disease. In: Fauci AS, Braunwald E, Isselbacker KJ, Wilson JD, Martin JB, et al, eds. *Harrison's principles of internal medicine*. New York: McGraw Hill, 1998:258-62.
3 Del Mar C, Jewell D. Tracking down the evidence. In: Silagy C, Haines A, eds. *Evidence based practice in primary care*. London: BMJ Publishing, 1998:21-33.
4 Sackett DL, Richardson WS, Rosenberg W, Haynes RB. *Evidence-based medicine*. London: Pearson Professional Publishing, 1997.
5 Ritchie CD, Bevan EA, Collier SJ. Importance of occult haematuria found at screening. *BMJ* 1986;292:681-3.
6 Hiatt RA, Ordonez JD. Dipstick urinalysis screening, asymptomatic microhematuria, and subsequent urological cancers in a population-based sample. *Cancer Epidemiol Biomarkers Prev* 1994;3:439-43.
7 Froom P, Gross M, Froom J, Caine Y, Margaliot S, Benbassat J. Factors associated with microhematuria in asymptomatic young men. *Clin Chem* 1986;32:2013-5.

(Accepted 19 April 1999)

Evidence based case report
Chlamydia infection in general practice

N R Hicks, M Dawes, M Fleminger, D Goldman, J Hamling, L J Hicks

Directorate of
Public Health and
Health Policy,
Oxfordshire Health
Authority, Oxford
OX3 7LG
N R Hicks,
consultant

Hollow Way
Medical Centre,
Oxford OX4 2NJ
M Dawes,
general practitioner
M Fleminger,
general practitioner
D Goldman,
general practitioner
J Hamling,
general practitioner
L J Hicks,
general practitioner

Correspondence to:
Dr N R Hicks
nicholas.hicks@
dphpc.ox.ac.uk

BMJ 1999;318:790–2

How common is chlamydia infection, and who should be investigated and treated for it? Is the net benefit of investigation worth the cost? At a recent discussion in our general practice it soon became apparent that our views and practices varied widely. Was there any evidence to help us reach a consensus? We resolved to try and find out.

Case report

Ms A, a 20 year old secretary, was worried because she had had vaginal discharge and irritation for three days. The discharge was slight, clear, watery, and non-offensive, and she had no abnormal vaginal bleeding. Ms A had changed her sexual partner two months previously. Soon after this she had contracted genital thrush, which responded to topical clotrimazole. She uses a combined contraceptive pill and does not use condoms. Ms A has no other sexual partners, and thinks it unlikely her partner has. However, she has little knowledge of his previous sexual history.

The only noteworthy finding at vaginal examination was that Ms A's cervix bled easily when swabbed. A high vaginal swab was taken from the posterior fornix, and two swabs were taken from the endocervix and the urethra—a standard cotton swab and a plastic shafted chlamydia swab respectively. Ms A was prescribed doxycycline (200 mg for seven days) and metronidazole (400 mg three times daily for seven days).

A few days later the laboratory reported that chlamydia had been detected. Ms A was invited back to the surgery and was upset to be told that she might have had a sexually transmitted disease. She and her partner were referred to the local sexually transmitted diseases clinic for further investigation and follow up.

Our uncertainty

The case of Ms A prompted discussion in the practice about who we should investigate and treat for chlamydia. Of course, we all wanted to prevent our patients suffering avoidable morbidity—for example, pelvic inflammatory disease, infertility, and ectopic pregnancy—and we also wanted to use the NHS's scarce resources as wisely as possible. But some of us thought there was no place for chlamydia investigation in primary care, arguing that as chlamydia tests were expensive and insensitive, patients should be treated for chlamydia whenever this organism was suspected clinically. Others felt it important to obtain a microbiological diagnosis wherever possible, and, as chlamydial infection can be asymptomatic, thought we should be searching for asymptomatic cases—for example, among sexually active women attending for cervical smears or for contraceptive advice. However, none of us knew how common chlamydia was in our practice, nor were we certain that treating an asymptomatic infection reduced subsequent morbidity. We did not know the magnitude of any benefits and harms associated with proactive case finding or whether any net benefit would be worth the resources consumed.

Search for evidence

It is frequently written that the first step in evidence based practice is to turn the clinical problem into an answerable question.[1] This proved more difficult than we first thought, as we wanted answers to several questions:
- Is genital chlamydia an important cause of clinically important morbidity?
- Does antibiotic treatment reduce subsequent morbidity in asymptomatic, sexually active women infected with chlamydia?
- If so, is case finding in our population likely to be a cost effective way of reducing clinically important morbidity?

Easy access
In the past, we might first have looked to standard textbooks for our answers. However, textbooks held in libraries are now more difficult to access from general practitioners' homes and surgeries than are online electronic databases. In addition, traditional textbooks are rarely written in a way that is sufficiently transparent to enable readers to determine how the authors reached their conclusions. More worryingly, the opinions expressed in textbooks may either be out of date even before publication or inconsistent with valid and relevant evidence.[2] We therefore decided to

> **Summary points**
>
> Chlamydia infection is the commonest treatable sexually transmitted disease in the United Kingdom; it is most common in sexually active women aged under 20
>
> Serological studies suggest that chlamydial infection may account for a large proportion of cases of tubal infertility and ectopic pregnancy
>
> 60-80% of genital chlamydia infections in women may be asymptomatic
>
> In one randomised trial, screening high risk women and treating those found to be infected reduced the incidence of pelvic inflammatory disease by about half in 12 months
>
> Access to the internet allows valid, relevant information to be identified and retrieved quickly—but appraising the evidence and deciding how best to reflect it in practice takes considerably longer

look for answers to our questions using the information we could access from home or the surgery.

Categories of evidence

We thought our questions were unlikely to be original. Similar questions ought to have been addressed by anyone drafting evidence based guidelines. We also thought that a great many original research papers would have been published about chlamydia, and that it would be an inappropriate use of our time to attempt to obtain, read, and appraise every relevant article. We therefore decided to search for recent systematic reviews about chlamydia; evidence based guidelines about the detection and treatment of chlamydia; and randomised controlled trials of treatment or case finding, or both, and treatment of asymptomatic chlamydia published after the most recent systematic review or evidence based guideline that we retrieved. NRH offered to spend up to one hour searching at home for relevant material using a computer connected to the internet.

Where to search?

Before searching, NRH checked the one relevant textbook he had at home.[3] It did not answer our questions. The next stops were Best Evidence[4] and the Cochrane Library,[5] searching with the single word "chlamydia." The search of Best Evidence identified five articles, none of which had promising titles. The Cochrane Library search produced two completed Cochrane reviews, both about chlamydia in pregnancy, and three reviews listed on the Database of Abstracts of Reviews of Effectiveness. None of these looked relevant, so the next step was the internet.

Controlled trials

The first stop was *Bandolier's* home page (www.jr2.ox.ac.uk/bandolier/). A search using "chlamydia" rapidly led to the full text of an article on treatment of chlamydia.[6] This article noted that the Centers for Communicable Disease in the United States had recently changed its recommended treatment for chlamydial infection from oral doxycycline (100 mg twice daily for 7 days) to a single dose (1 g) of azithromycin.[7] *Bandolier* had searched Medline for trials comparing doxycycline with azithromycin in the treatment of symptomatic and asymptomatic genital chlamydia and confirmed that both were effective treatments.

Bandolier had also looked at cost effectiveness, and it concluded that although azithromycin was more expensive, if compliance were better the higher drug costs would probably be "offset by lower costs associated with pelvic inflammatory disease, chronic pelvic pain, ectopic pregnancy, and tubal infertility." Perhaps the most startling information in this article, however, was the epidemiological data: chlamydia is the commonest curable bacterial sexually transmitted disease in the United Kingdom and the organism is most likely to be isolated in sexually active women under the age of 20 years, with rates in excess of 350 per 100 000 population (0.35%).

Recent guidelines and systematic reviews

The next step was to search for recent guidelines and systematic reviews. Medline Express for 1996, 1997, and January-March 1998 was searched with WinSpirs.

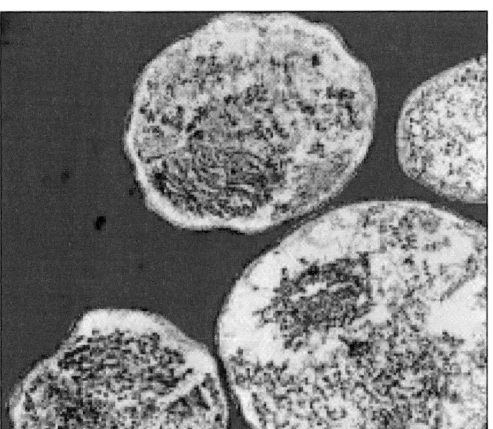

Chlamydia trachomatis: the cause of the commonest treatable sexually transmitted disease in the United Kingdom

A search for the medical subject heading (MeSH) term "chlamydia" in all subheadings produced 813 articles. This search was then limited by publication type to "meta-analysis" (1 article), "guideline" (2), "review academic" (5), "review" (83), and "randomised controlled trial" (10). Browsing the titles showed that one of the guidelines had been prepared by the Canadian Task Force on the Periodic Health Examination,[8] which has a reputation for using a rigorous approach based on systematic evidence to developing guidelines. The full text of the guideline is available free on the world wide web (www.cma.ca/cmaj/vol-154/1631.htm).

Canadian task force review

This text cited 201 references. In using a systematic approach to reviewing published reports and developing its recommendations it had considered many of the questions to which we sought answers. The text reported that in North America, as in Britain, chlamydia is the commonest sexually transmitted disease, and is two to three times as common as gonorrhoea. As in Britain, infection is most prevalent among sexually active women aged 15 to 19 years. In six Canadian studies, 1-25% of women tested were infected. Other risk factors and indicative signs were multiple sexual partners, a new partner in the previous year, no barrier method of contraception, low socioeconomic status, intermenstrual bleeding, cervical friability, and purulent cervical discharge. However, 60-80% of infections in women are asymptomatic. But what startled us most was the statement supported by 18 references that "serologic studies suggest that at least 64% of cases of tubal infertility, and 42% of ectopic pregnancies are attributable to chlamydial infection." Unfortunately, the guideline authors did not comment on the strength of inference that could be drawn from these 18 papers.

Does case finding reduce morbidity?

But was there any evidence that case finding and treating asymptomatic infection reduced morbidity? The guideline authors could identify only one controlled study in a non-pregnant population. The reference cited a paper presented to the International Symposium on Human Chlamydial Infections, which was unlikely to be retrievable quickly and cheaply. However, scanning the 10 randomised trials that had been identified from Medline indicated that the same study had been published later in the *New England Journal of Medicine*.[9] This article was readily retrieved the next day from the hospital library. (It could have been retrieved that night from online access to the BMA Library.)

The article reported a randomised controlled trial conducted in Seattle, in which 2607 asymptomatic women were randomised to an invitation to investigation for chlamydial infection (cervical swabs sent for enzyme linked immunosorbent assay and culture) and treatment if positive or to a control group given the "usual care." Women were followed for 12 months. The chlamydial infection rate in control women was 7%. The rate of clinically defined pelvic inflammatory disease in the 12 months after randomisation was reduced by 56% (relative risk 0.44, 95% confidence interval 0.20 to 0.90) in the intervention group compared with the control women. The absolute risk reduction was 1.1%; 2% of the control group developed pelvic inflammatory disease during follow up compared with 0.9% of the women in the intervention group. In other words, in Seattle, 91 sexually active women aged 18-34 years had to be invited for investigation for chlamydia to prevent one case of pelvic inflammatory disease. The study did not provide information about the impact of case finding on tubal damage, ectopic pregnancy, or infertility. Nor did it comment on any harm that may have resulted—for example, from treating women whose results were falsely positive, from mistaken reassurance of women given false negative results, or from the social implications of being told that one has an asymptomatic sexually transmitted disease. Nevertheless, we thought that this was an important study.

Studies in British general practice

But was the prevalence of chlamydia likely to be as high as 7% among any readily identifiable groups of our patients? We wanted some prevalence data from British general practice. Among the reviews identified on Medline was an article with a promising title.[10] This article cited nine prevalence studies of chlamydial infection undertaken in British general practices. The prevalence of infection ranged from 2% among asymptomatic women aged 15-40 attending for a cervical smear in Fife, Scotland, to 12% among women aged 16-44 requesting termination of pregnancy in inner city east London. The prevalence was also 12% among the mainly social class 3 women aged 19-58 attending for a cervical smear in an inner city Glasgow practice, and it was 11% in premenopausal women undergoing a speculum examination for any reason in a central London general practice.

What we learned and decided

Chlamydia is a much more important public health issue than any of us had suspected. We were all surprised at just how common it can be among young, sexually active women. We were also surprised that serological studies suggest that chlamydia may account for at least two thirds of tubal infertility and nearly half of ectopic pregnancies. Furthermore, we were impressed with the randomised controlled trial from Seattle which showed that in women in whom the

prevalence of chlamydial infection was 7%, inviting them for investigation and treatment where necessary reduced the rate of pelvic inflammatory disease by half in 12 months. This suggested to us that much of the morbidity caused by chlamydia may be preventable.

The evidence that we have seen did not allow us to identify unequivocally a single best practice for deciding in whom and how to investigate and treat chlamydia. Given that there is substantial geographical variation in chlamydia prevalence, we think that it is unlikely that a case finding policy can be devised that is equally cost effective for all practices in the United Kingdom. However, the data do suggest that systematic case finding and treatment of chlamydia could reduce potentially life-ruining morbidity for appreciable numbers of British women. Thus, we have decided that in the absence of national guidance we want to discuss and agree a way forward with other local practices, genitourinary physicians, microbiologists, gynaecologists, family planning clinics, and the health authority. One important next step might be to measure the prevalence of chlamydia infection in selected groups of our practice populations.

What about Ms A? We now know that she had several risk factors for chlamydia—she was young, sexually active, had a new sexual partner, and had a friable cervix. We should therefore have suspected chlamydia infection. Until there is a local guideline, we have agreed that whenever we suspect chlamydia we will offer to take chlamydia swabs and treat with doxycycline—unless compliance may be a problem, in which case we will use azithromycin. We will also refer patients and their partners to the genitourinary medicine clinic.

Although the evidence we found did not answer our questions completely it was the best evidence that we could find. We could not escape making a decision about what to do for our patients, as to do nothing would be a decision in itself. Our search took less than an hour plus a 10 minute trip to the library. Reading and discussing the material we retrieved took rather longer, perhaps three hours. We learned a lot and made a decision about patient management that is based on the best evidence we could find. We think that our time was well spent.

Competing interests: NRH has received lecture fees for speaking at postgraduate education meetings for general practitioners sponsored by the manufacturers of azithromycin.

1 Sackett DL, Richardson WS, Rosenberg W, Haynes RB. *Evidence-based medicine—how to practice and teach EBM.* London: Churchill Livingstone, 1997.
2 Antman EM, Lau J, Kupelnick B, Mosteller F, Chalmers TC. A comparison of results of meta-analyses of randomised controlled trials and recommendations of clinical experts. *JAMA* 1992;268:240-8.
3 McPherson A, ed. *Women's problems in general practice.* 3rd ed. Oxford: Oxford University Press, 1992. (Oxford General Practice Series 24.)
4 American College of Physicians. *Best evidence: linking medical research to practice 1997* [CD Rom]. Philadelphia: American College of Physicians, 1997.
5 *The Cochrane Library* [database on disc and CD Rom]. Cochrane Collaboration; 1997, 1997 Issue 4. Oxford: Update Software, 1997.
6 Chalmydial STD treatment. *Bandolier* 1996;3(28):4-6. (http://www.jr2.ox.ac.uk/bandolier/band28/b28-4.html)
7 Levine WC, Berg AO, Johnson RE, Rolfe RT, Stone KM, Hook EW III, et al. Development of sexually transmitted diseases treatment guidelines 1993. *Sex Transm Dis* 1994;21(suppl):96-101.
8 Davies HD, Wang EE. Periodic health examination, 1996 update: 2. Screening for chlamydial infections. Canadian Task Force on the Periodic Health Examination. *Can Med Assoc J* 1996;154;1631-44.
9 Scholes D, Stergachis A, Heidrich MD, Andrilla H, Holmes KK, Stamm WG. Prevention of pelvic inflammatory disease by screening for cervical chlamydial infection. *N Engl J Med* 1996;334:1362-6.
10 Stokes T. Screening for chlamydia in general practice: a literature review and summary of the evidence. *J Public Health Med* 1997;19:222-32.

(Accepted 2 September 1998)

129

Index

Page numbers in **bold** type refer to figures, those in *italics* refer to tables or boxed material.